RAISING SOUND SLEEPERS

Helping Children Use their Senses to Rest and Self-Soothe

ADAM BLANNING MD

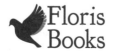

Floris
Books

First published by Floris Books in 2023
© 2023 Adam Blanning

Adam Blanning has asserted his right under the
Copyright, Design and Patents Act 1988
to be identified as the Author of this Work

 Also available as an eBook

British Library CIP Data available
ISBN 978-178250-842-7
Printed & bound by MBM Print SCS Ltd, Glasgow

 Floris Books supports sustainable forest
management by printing this book on
Forest Stewardship Council® certified paper

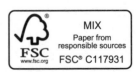

MIX
Paper from
responsible sources
FSC® C117931
FSC
www.fsc.org

CONTENTS

INTRODUCTION

How do you know when to actively guide a child's development and when to trust in the process? That is a challenging and recurring question for every parent. Fortunately, most aspects of child development unfold out of an innate wisdom. You don't need to have read a parenting book to teach your child to walk, because children naturally seek that experience of being upright and they know what to do. That process of naturally moving towards new skills holds true for many aspects of development. But sleep and soothing unfold in their own special way. Coming to rest seems like it should be the most natural process in the world, but in many ways it is a learned skill. While some children learn to self-soothe without fuss or frustration and find what they need, many of today's children seem to struggle to settle and feel calm.

Part of the challenge of raising sound sleepers surely comes from the fact that we are born into a world that routinely drowns us in images and sounds. The outside stimulation offered by our modern society provides a rich but very narrow and intense sensory palate. We are continually prompted to react and pay attention to the outside world. For many children, outer impressions so saturate their consciousness that they don't have enough space to even sense their inner world. Without that inward connection they easily feel overwhelmed and unsettled. Young children's lack of an inner anchor makes balancing and navigating the demands of the outside world a challenge. Our inner world tells us many important messages about our well-being. Being able to hear those messages makes the journey through childhood, and through all of life, easier.

Fortunately, there are dependable, observable steps each person can take to connect to this quieter, more regenerative part of our physiology. The pathway towards our inner world is inside all of us, even if we sometimes lose our connection to it in the face of so many other louder, faster external demands.

The first steps on this inward pathway are provided to babies already at birth, but processes for self-soothing necessarily evolve as children grow into more independent activity. Children weave back and forth between courageous outer exploration and the need for greater inward security. Most measures of child development miss this inward aspect. They take careful note of the (outer) milestones for gross and fine motor skills, and for speech and socialization, but there is little, if any, discussion about the inner steps also needed for growth.

> For each developmental step of outward physical and social exploration, a reciprocal step towards greater self-soothing and inner sensing also needs to be taken.

There are, in fact, a whole series of developmental 'milestones' for achieving rest. Individual children work through these steps of self-soothing with variable timing and dynamics, but each child must practice them. They provide the foundation for resilience in the face of outer stress.

Parents, teachers, caregivers and healthcare providers can all benefit from learning about these steps for self-soothing. Why? Because children who get lost along this inner pathway often experience emotional dysregulation and social insecurity. Patterns of separation anxiety, disrupted sleep, restless agitation, repeated interruptions or provocative behaviors, as well as a wide range of self-stimulating and even addictive patterns, can all relate to a blocked step on this developmental journey. These kinds of behaviors commonly signify a disturbed connection to one's own sense of well-being. Conversely, learning to connect to our own body, to turn inward, and to understand our own needs, helps each of us, in turn, feel more 'comfortable in our skin'.

The goal of this book is to help you learn about the major steps along this inner pathway for self-soothing, and how those steps can be strengthened by offering your child healthy sensory experiences and by learning more about key developmental transitions during childhood. This will empower your parenting. It will help you see and respond to the needs of your child. Working with this inner pathway has proven helpful for families who are struggling to find healthy sleep patterns, or who are seeking better ways to parent a very anxious child.

Let observation be your guide

The descriptions in this book come from closely observing many children – hundreds, even thousands. Each time, the main task was to try and understand, 'What do you really need?' Some insights have come through personal parenting experiences, like trying to put a very tired child to bed. That can be an arduous task admittedly, but sometimes it brings a moment of clarity. One such moment came when one of my own children, fatigued to the point of complete meltdown, said while getting into bed, 'I want, I want, I want... (dramatic pause) ...I want nothing!' This was so true, and what a wonderful revelation! It meant that there was nothing more from the outside that was going to help – not a drink of water, a kind word, a gentle reassurance, or a hug. Not even an 'I love you.' All that was needed was for her to be left alone so that she could relax, let go of the outside world, and find her own place of rest. It brought a small pang of parenting sorrow because, at that moment, whether or not she felt good was beyond my control. That shadow quickly passed and was replaced with relief because, instead of desperately trying to solve her distress, it was possible to just step back and provide the space she needed to calm and self-soothe. She needed to inwardly sense what she needed, which she did. In moments she was asleep. That was a valuable, early lesson about giving a child permission to practice their own quieting process.

Many related experiences have reinforced the importance of that lesson, especially through seeing how different kinds of children self-soothe. Good opportunities come through my work as a developmental consultant for schools. This is a unique task as a physician, one which involves quietly observing from the back of a classroom and looking to see why a particular child acts a certain way. One frequent concern of teachers is the continually disruptive child. There are, of course, many reasons why a child may disrupt a class – fatigue, confusion, boredom, impulsivity – but there is one special pattern you can learn to recognize. It is when a child experiences a kind of lonely disorientation and then acts out. This particular behavior usually comes when things are getting quieter in the classroom and there is less outside sensory input, such as when a class listens to a song or story, or when a child is asked to enter into independent activity like drawing or writing. As a quiet observer you can literally watch how some children become unmoored and don't quite know what they should be doing, so they do something provocative. They yell, they poke, they act wild or talk in a strange voice, all with the goal of gaining outside attention. After they have provoked the attention of the teacher and/or the other students, the child immediately feels more secure and grounded. It does not seem to matter so much if the attention is negative. The goal is to find orientation through outer stimulus.

A variation of this same behavior comes during some medical appointments in my office, when a child will ask the parent a question about every three-and-a-half minutes. You can just about set your watch by it – the questioning reminds you of a sonar 'ping' meant to map just exactly how far away the parent is. Repeated 'sonar-type' questions ensure that the parent also won't forget about the child. The questions reinforce regular connection. The parent can't become too engaged in anything else. Both the disruptive child in the classroom and the child with a hundred questions during a medical visit usually share a strong reliance on the outside world for security and orientation.

An additional element has also become clearer. In many different conversations with both parents and teachers about children who tend to act this way, it emerges that these children almost always have a hard time falling asleep. Parents consistently report that bedtime is a long process and requires a lot of work to get the child to settle. Frequently, these children won't settle at all without a parent staying or lying right next to them. The children will fight to keep a parent there in the bed until they have fallen asleep. Then, if the child wakes up in the middle of the night and a parent isn't there, the child goes and finds the parent, so that either the child sleeps the rest of the night in the parent's bed, or the parent comes and sleeps in the child's bed. This way of seeking comfort is a natural part of childhood, but beyond a certain age the child's dependence on outer reassurance becomes problematic. They become stuck. Stepping back, we see that it is part of a constellation of behaviors in which a child must repeatedly turn to the outside to find guidance or reassurance. That behavior pattern suggests that the child needs, but is probably also struggling, to take the next steps in developing more independent capacities for calming and self-orientation.

How does this correlate with a child's daytime behavior? When a child consistently struggles to quiet and settle during the transition to sleep – which is actually the main time we practice the process of self-soothing each and every day – then it makes sense that the child may also feel disoriented with independent daytime tasks. The process of calming and self-orienting that needs to happen just before sleep is the same kind of process that we call on when we move from busy, outer social engagement to a more quiet, independent activity. In terms of self-orienting ability, it makes sense that if a child has not yet been able to develop reliable, self-soothing steps at night, then they may also show disruptive behaviors during waking hours. This pattern is also true for separation anxiety. As a physician working with many children, I have learned to always ask about sleep when there are behavioral challenges during the daytime, and ask about daytime separation anxiety whenever there are sleep challenges. The two very frequently go together.

> By actively helping children learn the next steps towards greater self-soothing and inward sensing, we can not only change stuck sleep patterns, but we can also bring a greater sense of security to a child's daytime social activities.

Another key insight is that through recognizing these connections we begin to see multiple types of challenging behaviors as more than just an annoyance. We begin to understand them as an honest expression of a child's needs

– their sensory needs, emotional needs, social needs – which can overlap. What is exciting is that we can work with each of these needs by strengthening a child's own calming capacities. Here are some examples:

★ **When a child insists that a parent lie next to them until they fall asleep.** This pattern usually relates to an incompletely developed sense of touch – a sensory need. Learn more about this in **Chapter 3: When Soothing Gets Stuck and How to Shift It.**

★ **Fighting any kind of separation** (even allowing time for a parent to go to the bathroom alone) often reflects a child's need for avoiding experiences of loneliness and isolation – an emotional need. Learn more about this in **Chapter 4: Finding Balance from Age 1 Onward.**

★ **Constant questions or continual arguing** frequently represent a child's desperate need to feel connection – a social need for orientation. Learn more about this in **Chapter 7: Independence and Boundaries from Age 2½ Onward.**

★ **A bedtime dash through the house,** paradoxical as it may seem, can in fact be a way for a child to quiet the mind and find more rest. Learn more about this in **Chapter 8: Building Well-being and Resilience for All Ages.**

Recognizing these behaviors as *needs*, not problems, is the first step. The second step is to learn about the individual 'soothing milestones' that make up the inner pathway towards greater self-orientation and calming. The third step is to then gather the tools and experiences that will support a developmental step forward – a courageous step towards a new capacity. With these three steps we can help children learn to self-soothe, rest, sleep soundly and enhance their sense of well-being.

1. WHAT IS THE INNER SENSORY PATHWAY?

To start this exploration we must first expand our picture of how children sense the world. We need to open our awareness to the more subtle ways in which children (and adults) sense and orient themselves. This helps us build a more holistic understanding of child development.

When we think of the senses, we usually think of vision, hearing, taste, smell and touch. These five senses are the main 'windows' for taking in perceptions of the outside world. They guide us on a daily basis, conveying essential impressions and information. But in truth, they stand only in the middle of a much broader spectrum of sensory activity. For beyond this boundary realm of 'outside-meets-inside', we reach both further into ourselves (as part of a process of self-perception and self-regulation) and further out towards other people (to gain a deeper understanding of them). We rely on these 'extended' sensing activities to guide us on a daily basis, even if their messages are less obvious. In order to acknowledge these sensing activities, which will be described in the following paragraphs, we must increase the number of senses we pay attention to beyond the traditional five.

A core aspect of this expanded sensory view is not just that there are a greater number of senses, but also that the senses have particular relationships with one other. They stand in a specific arrangement, ordered because of their specific dynamics. A full spectrum of sensory activities extends from our own inward-most sensing of health and well-being – which we can call our sense of well-being – to our most outwardly directed, social striving to perceive the essence of another human being – which we can call the 'I' sense. The pathway between perceiving the state of our own innermost world and the highly individual qualities and characteristics of another person encompasses a very full range of sensing activities – twelve main ones in total – and together they form an archway of connection and orientation:

Outer-world sensing   Inner-world sensing

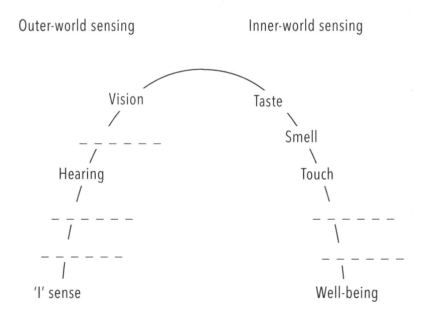

This is admittedly a different way of learning about our senses, though medically and educationally it's become clear that recognizing only five senses is not adequate. You will see that the archway is incomplete – I've left some spaces to fill in. For example, where is our sense of balance? How do we account for our capacities for social sensing? There are holes in the more traditional understanding of five main senses. Fortunately, this kind of expanded view of the human being has been successfully researched and explored as a part of holistic educational, remedial and medical initiatives around the world. The task of this book is to take some of the fruits of that work, and show how it can support better rest, sleep, self-soothing and resilience in children.

Rather than taking this sensory spectrum at face value, let's work to build this expanded sensory bridge through some simple observations.

Identifying additional senses beyond the classic five is not so difficult. For example, we all experience our sense of balance whenever we bend over, stand up too quickly, ride an escalator, or reach for a high object. Balance is clearly distinct from hearing, vision, smell, taste or touch. This adds a sixth sense.

Neurologists and physical and occupational therapists also highlight the importance of our sense of proprioception. Proprioception is the knowledge of where our limbs are in space without needing to look and see what we are doing. Through proprioception we feel the position and activity of our joints. That sensing capacity can actually be enlarged to describe a whole sense of feeling oneself in movement.

We will explore these two senses in much more detail in the coming chapters. The addition of balance and movement (or proprioception) makes seven senses, plus our own inner sense of well-being and our outer 'I' sense makes nine senses.

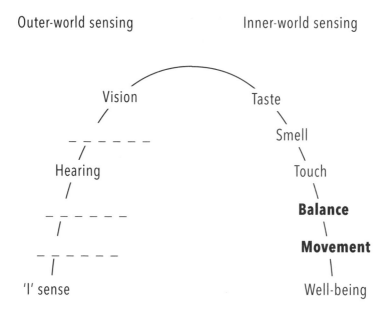

Outer-world sensing   Inner-world sensing

Vision   Taste

Smell

Hearing   Touch

Balance

Movement

'I' sense   Well-being

The addition of those two senses completes an arc of connection from outward sensing (vision) to inward sensing (well-being). The half of the arc that is more inwardly directed plays a crucial role in the life of all young children. We will focus on these six steps for the majority of this book. But for completeness, let's briefly describe the outwardly focused sensory pathway.

The outwardly focused pathway plays a much bigger role in the life of older children and adults, standing behind capacities like language development, abstract thought, the reading of social cues and even moral perception and judgement of other people. That half of the sensory arc deserves a book of its own, but here we will merely outline them.

There are three empty slots.

The first missing sense is perhaps taken for granted, even though it is quite familiar. It's the capacity we carry for sensing warmth. We are most conscious of it when we perceive the temperature of an outer object through our skin, so warmth is commonly thrown in with the sense of touch. Touch and warmth, however, are separate sensory activities, even though each is experienced at the boundary of our body. Research studies show that a person's sensitivity of touch does not necessarily correlate with the activity of their warmth perception[1] and, interestingly, that there are neurological overlaps between our sensing of physical warmth and our perception of social or moral warmth.[2] We therefore need to identify a distinct sensory capacity for warmth.

The second gap is for sensing the meaning of a word, while the third is for sensing a thought. One only needs to communicate with other people, especially in a language that is not one's mother tongue, to appreciate that hearing sounds is not the same as understanding words. And even in one's own language there are frequently times when we might understand all the words a person speaks, but not be able to comprehend their thoughts. Hearing sounds, identifying a word and understanding a thought are distinct capacities. When we combine these steps together, we see that to truly perceive another person we must first be interested in them (an aspect of the sense of warmth), we must listen (hearing), attend to what they are saying (word), and work to understand what they are thinking (thoughts). Hopefully, we can then gain some true perception of their individual self (I). These are only very brief indications about this outwardly oriented arc of sensory activity, but they mark important points along the pathway for truly meeting another human being.[3]

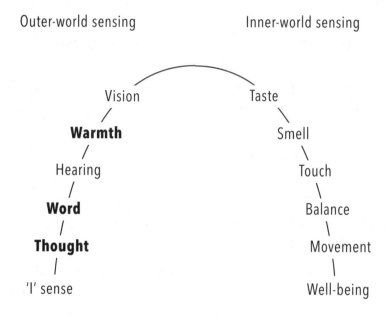

This constellation of twelve senses as a continuum from inside to outside world, was first recognized and described by Rudolf Steiner, an Austrian philosopher, educator and scientist, who developed a body of work that has laid the foundation for Waldorf education, Camphill schools, and anthroposophic medicine. His first major task as an adult, after completing his university studies, was to work as a private tutor for the family of a child with profound developmental delays. The child could not speak and barely interacted with his environment, but over years of intensive, individualized care and education he improved dramatically. By the time he was a young adult he was able to attend university, study medicine and become a physician.

We are blessed with the fruit of Steiner's intensive observation and study. Working with a whole spectrum of senses, from inside to outside, allows us to see fine shades of developmental growth and maturation. The background story of Steiner's remarkably successful effort to help a child with developmental challenges should rouse our curiosity. What more can we learn from this? How can we become wiser in our observations? What new insights will come?

From personal experience I can share that this sensory progression was not completely obvious when I first encountered it. I learned about it as part of my own search for a more holistic approach to medicine. Probably part of the reason it felt a little inaccessible was that I had worked hard to perform well in a medical environment that focuses mostly on nouns (anatomic structures, lab results, drug compounds). I had not had as much practice learning to think about health and development through more dynamic processes and spectrums, though it was exciting to know that it was possible! This circle of the senses offered a doorway into understanding children's behaviors in a whole new way.

Then a couple of threads wove together. As a physician, I've always been very interested in children and how they learn and thrive, and so I set up a small, private medical practice where I could focus more on the living dynamics of health and illness. I needed my own, protected place to think in new ways. As a result, I stopped my work teaching family medicine at a medical school. That shift was also motivated by the opportunity to stay home several days a week with my own young children and care for them from infancy to kindergarten. Those years helped bridge theoretical knowledge with practical experience. So when I describe the magical stage when a child stops crying after being handed to their mother who *smells* like milk (but the child doesn't actually *taste* a drop of milk), that's because I saw this distinct activity of smell versus taste being demonstrated. Likewise, I've experienced the point when *touch* becomes a powerful way to soothe, when, as a non-nursing parent (who didn't *smell* like milk and certainly couldn't produce it), a new doorway opened for calming my children. Piece by piece, Steiner's description of the inner sensory pathway started to make sense. Those differentiations of taste, smell, and touch play a tremendous role in the life of babies and are the focus of Chapter 2.

In my professional life, I began teaching early childhood teachers as well as other doctors interested in child development, and whenever I described this self-soothing pathway they got excited. Teachers started exploring it in their classrooms, and it gave them new tools for working with students who frequently disrupt or seem stuck on challenging behaviors like thumb-sucking, or even self-stimulating (masturbation) behaviors during nap time (we will consider those last two behaviors in Chapter 9). The teachers saw good results.

Next came opportunities to observe how teenagers and adults also use this pathway to calm and orient themselves whenever the outside world feels unpredictable, and how children with developmental challenges consistently invoke these sensory pathways to anchor themselves. Even post-traumatic patterns and certain kinds of addictions became more understandable by observing and working with these steps of soothing and self-perception. But the most consistent and practical application has been working with families who wish to help their children feel calmer, improve their sleep patterns and develop greater resilience.

And so we will start by looking at how this inner sensory pathway relates to soothing right from the beginning of life.

2. SOOTHING PATTERNS FOR BABIES

The process of calming, orienting and soothing begins right after birth. It plays a huge role in the life of every infant and stands as a core part of early learning and development. Babies are gifted with some key aspects of that process right away. Then, gradually, they add more tools to expand their soothing repertoire. In this chapter we will explore the senses of taste, smell and touch. They greatly contribute to the processes of self-soothing and calming in the first year but play different roles, and enter into a child's experience, at different times. There is a beautiful mirroring that happens here, for as children grow stronger and become increasingly aware of the surrounding world, more inward-soothing pathways open up to them, which provide a calming anchor for when the outside world becomes too busy, too overwhelming, or when they are too tired. The first year of life is full of such adjustments and transitions.

The biggest shift we experience in our whole lifetime is probably birth. In a short period of time babies go from a quiet, warm, floating experience in which awareness of any outside activity is muted and soft, to abrupt, new, dramatic sensations of cold, touch, light, sound, and gravity. What a change! It is certainly a shock and requires all kinds of adaptation. It's no wonder that infants are only awake for very short periods of time. Their fluctuations of waking and sleeping are a kind of developmental 'stutter-step' – awake for a while, then sleeping to recover, then awake for a little while longer. It takes years for a child to become used to being in the world, and they may not be ready to face a full day of activity without naps until kindergarten age.

So what helps to calm and orient children during such a vital transitional period? How do they manage to make such dramatic shifts at birth and not become completely overwhelmed? Right from the start they are given a gift that helps to soothe and calm them. It is the sweet taste of milk.

The sense of taste

Whether an infant experiences distress from fatigue, disorientation, hunger or physical discomfort, nursing makes it better. It is a universal balm. That happens because our pathway to an enhanced state of well-being begins with the sense of taste. Gentle touch and attention are also part of an infant's experience of being nursed, but it is the taste of milk that is vital. We know that because a baby is calmed when it tastes milk from the breast or from a bottle, calmed whether it takes in donated milk or formula. The taste of milk makes every new baby feel secure.

This connection between taste and an enhanced experience of well-being is not limited to infancy. As human beings, we celebrate special occasions with taste. We nurture the ones we love with taste when we cook a meal or provide treats, and we self-medicate with taste when we eat for comfort. There is a consistent connection between our sense of taste (especially for sweet foods or flavors) and self-soothing. That's a great gift, built into us from the beginning. Taste connects us to our inner world and creates a buffer against all that is going on outside of us. Eat a piece of chocolate or some other nice treat and see if this is not true! Feed a hungry child and the child feels better, not just because of the nutrients or an increase in blood sugar, but because taste calms. The sensory process of tasting brings a subtle reorientation, turning us more towards our inner world, which makes us feel more whole. Taste is the first, foundational pathway for feeling soothed and connecting back to our inner world.

We can summarize the relationship this way:

Taste >>> Well-being

Even though taste is built into our experience from birth, it evolves and grows. A child's first experiences of taste are provided predominantly from the outside; they are almost entirely receptive. But during the first year of life, children adapt and extend their 'tasting' activities so that they are not just about nutrition but also orientation. Children often start that shift by finding a thumb or finger to suck on. Then, once they can crawl around the room, children put all kinds of objects in their mouth. The mouth begins to function not just as a taste organ but also as a broader organ for exploration. What starts as a strictly receptive process for calming broadens into a larger sensory interaction with the world.

That's a first important developmental insight: children are innately provided with pathways for soothing, which, in time, they expand, explore, and make their own.

The sense of smell

A second important developmental insight is that children diversify their pathways for soothing, usually with predictable patterns. We can see this with the sense of smell.

New parents quickly learn to appreciate the connection between taste and soothing. Taste is indeed *the* great balm for the transition from the security of the womb. But it would be a tremendous burden if we were solely reliant on taste for all our self-soothing over the whole of a lifetime – we would have to be continuously fed every time we felt worried, confused, experienced pain, or needed to fall asleep.

Instead, we learn to diversify our pathways for soothing. Rather than remaining reliant on taste as we grow stronger and adapt to the conditions of the outside world, we learn to be comforted by smell.

You can observe this shift at about a month or 6 weeks of age. At that point an infant will already begin to quiet just with the smell of milk, even before having tasted anything.

Anticipation is part of this calming, of course, but smell brings its own soothing power.

Fathers and non-nursing parents learn the reality of the soothing power of smell pretty quickly. This happens when their child – who was so worried and upset, fussing and not responding to anything offered – suddenly stops crying as soon as they are handed back to the parent who smells like milk. Sometimes tears are still rolling down the child's cheeks as anguish fades and a beautiful smile appears. Smell has brought calm; no nursing is required, just smell. It's a kind of soothing magic.

Taste and smell are both doorways for engaging with the outside environment, but in relation to the full arc of the twelve senses, they both orient us more inwardly. To experience a taste or smell, a substance must enter our inner space through the mouth or nose. Both experiences are mediated by the activity of sensory receptors at the boundary of our body, but their effects are not the same. Smell affects us more deeply; it is more visceral and takes us a step further into our inner world.

For example, consider how deeply our sense of smell connects to our memory: the associations that come with the scent of baking, or of a wood fire, or of a loved one's shampoo. Such associations evoke strong impressions in us, and right from an early age they help to anchor us.

Children know a lot about the sense of smell and its connection to comfort. Many children like to have beloved blankets, dolls and stuffed animals because they act as comfort 'anchors'. They soothe a child not just because of how they feel or look, but also because of how they smell. Watch a child take their favorite teddy bear or quilt and see how, as they squeeze, hug and embrace it, they also inhale its smell. They nuzzle right in. And children often do not want to surrender their beloved item to be washed. That's instinctive wisdom because, even if it is very dirty and desperately needs to be cleaned, it is going to lose some of its distinctive smell.

This sensory connection of smell to well-being is, again, not limited to the first months of life. Children take comfort in the smell of a parent or other loved one long after the time for nursing has passed. Older children love to snuggle in, nose first. As teenagers, we may treasure the special smell of a boyfriend's or girlfriend's T-shirt. As adults, we can feel more relaxed with aromatherapy, or enjoy the smell of coffee even if we are not planning on drinking any. Just the scent changes how we feel and helps us be more grounded.

This greater 'inwardness' of smell also has its anatomical expression. The nerve bundles that transmit our sense of smell travel back into the brain more directly than just about any other sense experience. And the location of our smell receptors is more internal. You can't 'sip' or 'lick' a smell in the same way that you can reach out to taste something – smell has to come into you.

Taste calms and orients us; smell soothes us with a more intimate, more visceral quality. We can therefore place an additional element on the inward pathway of self-soothing:

Taste > **Smell** >>> Well-being

The sense of touch

The next sensing activity on this inward arc of connection may come as a surprise, even though it has already been mentioned – it is the sense of touch. We usually think of touch as being an outwardly directed activity, a way for us to know the *outer* world. But let's consider for a moment what Rudolf Steiner has to say about the sense of touch based on his own research:

> When you touch objects, you actually perceive only yourself. You touch an object and if it is hard it presses forcibly on you; if it is soft its pressure is only slight. You perceive nothing of the object, however; you sense only the effect upon yourself, the change in yourself. A hard object pushes your organs far back into you. You perceive this resistance as a change in your own organism when you perceive by the means of touch.[1]

This is a revolutionary statement! Our thinking about touch generally relates to the way we use skin contact to know the qualities of the outer world: how to grasp an object, how to cut with scissors, how to type on a keyboard. But we actually use touch to *perceive ourselves*. Children seek touch, long for touch, as a way to calm and orient themselves just for this reason. Touch experiences bring better awareness of boundary, of embodiment. That's why children love to be swaddled, held and hugged. As children grow stronger and become more mobile – pushing, lifting, squeezing the world around them – touch contributes not just to outward exploration but more fundamentally to the way they sense and know themselves.

Let's look at the first year of a child's life. What happens when the taste of milk or the smell of a parent is not enough to soothe an infant or toddler every time? At this point a new soothing 'doorway' opens through the sense of touch. Through being held, a child can be comforted not only by their parents but also by other loving adults, including non-nursing parents, grandparents, and other familiar caregivers. This provides new possibilities for calming and orienting.

Touch calms. Swaddling, patting and rubbing are familiar ways to help a child settle. A hug reassures them when there is a shock or a surprise, and it brings comfort when a child trips or bangs a knee. Rubbing or cradling a child's head when they have bumped it against something does little if anything to heal the injury itself, but the sensation of being touched provides solace. Touch helps a child feel their own boundary so that they can reorient and better feel themselves. Touch is actually one of the most important ways in which we support our own sense of well-being. This is not only true for children, it also applies to adult life, too.

What do you see when you walk into a room full of anxious people waiting for an unknown event or outcome? What are they doing? They are predictably invoking their own sense of touch. Because they don't know exactly what is going to happen next in the outer world, they are all working to perceive themselves, to feel their own boundary.

They sit on their hands, bite their fingernails, fold their arms, or repeatedly cross and uncross their legs. These are all ways that we intentionally (though perhaps unconsciously) stimulate our sense of touch.

Limited touch can result in less awareness of self. Children who spent their early lives in busy orphanages, where there was little experience of being held or touched by a caring adult, often show disturbed capacities for self-soothing and self-regulation.[2] They lacked the opportunity to feel their own body, to feel their own boundary, and to connect to themselves in this important way.

Yet there are paradoxes within the sense of touch. Loving touch often brings security, but unwelcome touch may feel invasive or aggressive. Both are true because touch stands at a unique place in the arc of the senses. It marks an important threshold between outer and inner. On the one hand, you need to come into contact with an outer object in order to have a sensation of touch. On the other, you cannot control how another person will respond to an experience of touch from the outside. We receive touch, but the experience of touch is mainly our own. To a great extent, children's reactions to touch depend upon their own process of perception. This becomes clearer if we compare it to the other senses.

Vision, for example, is quite different. Visual input comes completely from the outside. Our only real control of vision comes when we close our eyes or divert our gaze. Otherwise, we are wide open to our surrounding environment. That is why visual arts have such a profound effect: we are guided by the artist through a special sensory experience.

Tasting, too, comes from the outside: we need outside substance in order to taste. Individual variations influence what we like or do not like, but people go to the restaurants of world-class chefs for a reason – to be provided with a special taste experience.

Smell, which frequently brings strong emotional reactions and associations, also depends on the outside environment. The outside world must provide something for us to smell.

We can seek visual, gustatory (taste), and olfactory (smell) experiences, but we cannot create them ourselves. The sights, tastes and smells of dreams or hallucinations – which are altered types of consciousness – are not part of our true connection to the outside world.

With the sense of touch, however, we are more empowered. We can actively seek and create touch on our own.

Touch marks the place on the inward sensing pathway where we really begin to participate in our own soothing process. At the beginning of life we mainly receive touch. But as a child learns to roll, scoot, crawl, walk and toddle away from a parent, they simultaneously find more ways to touch through cuddling, rubbing, hugging and squeezing. That continues through the rest of life: we receive touch from the outside, but also seek and create touch experiences ourselves, whether we affectionately reach out to hug a loved one, or nervously rub our hands while awaiting an unknown outcome.

With this insight, we can make sense of the placement of touch on the pathway of inner sensing and connecting to a sense of well-being:

Taste > Smell > Touch >>> Well-being

The sense of vision

At the beginning of this chapter, I mentioned the wonderful mirroring that occurs between our progression along the inner sensory pathway and our increasing awareness of the surrounding world. Assuming that this sequenced progression does indeed have some validity, we might ask: if smell is a step more inward than taste, what would be a corresponding step outward towards the world around us?

Taking a step outwards from taste brings us to what we can think of as the most neutral activity of our senses: vision. Visual impressions do not impact us as directly as those of taste or smell do. How many objects do you encounter in your field of vision each day – thousands, hundreds of thousands, millions? How many of them do you consciously register? How many of them anchor you and help you feel calmer and more oriented? Probably not so many.

Vision can soothe us, but it more regularly pulls us outside of ourselves. When we see a beautiful sunset or concentrate to thread a needle we may become more still, but those are special circumstances. Visual impressions instead live in a realm of loose engagement. When we see the elements of vision – light, shadow, color – we quickly choose to focus and look more closely, or we dismiss the images and move on. We can direct our attention either inwards or outwards.

Through the activity of tasting, a little bit of the outside world enters our own domain. We meet a bit of the outside world and change it. We moisten, chew and dissolve the substance as we taste it and begin to break it down. Similarly, all the air we breathe in (through smell) changes. It is warmed and moistened. The very small particles of substance we sense through smell are carried in on that stream of warmed and moistened air. In contrast, we do not warm and moisten every object we look at, nor do we start to dissolve and break down everything in our visual field. Whether or not you look at an object has little recognizable effect on the physical qualities of that object. Our sense of sight holds a quite neutral space.

We can also ask: what is the role of vision in soothing and orienting for a very young child? The truth is that newborns' vision is quite blurry. Infants are only gradually able to focus on outside objects, and only those that are within a few feet of their face. Coordination of eye movements right after birth is poor. Vision takes time to achieve full development. It is not until a child reaches kindergarten or elementary school age that vision typically approaches 20/20.

A baby first begins to really see and respond to faces at around the same time that smell brings comfort. These two movements complement each other. As a child makes more connection to the outside world through vision, the sense of smell brings a reciprocal capacity for greater inward security and solace.

We have now established the first few 'stepping-stones' that lead from the sense of vision to the sense of well-being along the inner sensory pathway:

Outside world <<< Vision > Taste > Smell >
Touch >>> Well-being

Quick reminders

★ Children are guided by their sensory impressions. Taste, then smell, and eventually touch, serve as the foundational anchors for soothing in the first 6–12 months of life. They focus children's attention inwards, which is calming and orienting.

★ For each developmental step of exploration out into the world, children need to take reciprocal steps towards better calming and self-orienting (see Chapter 10 for more in-depth information about developmental stutter-steps).

★ Children's capacities to self-soothe and rest evolve with time. If your previously successful soothing routine suddenly seems to stop working, it probably means that your child is growing into a new developmental phase! (See Chapter 3 for more on this transition.)

Questions to consider

★ When does your child turn to taste or smell for soothing?

★ What are the stages or ages when these first steps on the inner sensory pathway (taste and smell) seem most helpful? Are there times when the process feels stuck and what does that look like? What happens when there is an over-reliance on only one sense experience to quiet and soothe?

★ Reflect on which practices you, as an adult, use to calm and focus yourself. What role do taste and smell play in your own life?

★ Where do you see your child turn to touch as a way to calm?

★ What role does touch play in your own adult life?

★ How was the process of learning to sleep and soothe for you, personally? Was it easy, anxious, fast, slow? What were your soothing anchors as a young child?

3. WHEN SOOTHING GETS STUCK AND HOW TO SHIFT IT

We will now explore how these 'stepping-stones' along the sensory pathway provide very practical help for families, teachers, and anyone who works therapeutically with children. Let's summarize three core ideas of this approach.

1. **You can take it with you.** While the world can feel overwhelming, unpredictable, and unsafe, this pathway reminds us that there are built-in developmental tools to support us. The more we explore these self-soothing capacities, the braver we can be in our outward explorations. As children find the physical strength and courage to freely explore the outside world, they also move naturally from being exclusively soothed from the outside (mainly by parents and caregivers) towards more inward possibilities for self-soothing.

> If you are going to travel farther and farther
> away from a parent, then you need to be able
> to take more and more of your feeling
> of security with you.

2. **There is no deadline.** Children learn to crawl
   without detailed instructions or bribes; they know
   it is the right thing to do. Similarly, just as many of
   the outer milestones for development follow a
   predictable rhythm, so too do children enter new
   stages of growth when they are ready to practice
   more independent self-soothing. It is better if we
   can recognize and meet this process of development
   as it unfolds naturally.

> There is a natural progression to this inward/
> outward learning, and we do not need to
> impose an artificial timeline on it.

3. **There will be stutter-steps.** The most common
   clue that a child is ready to make a shift along this
   inner pathway is **when the soothing method you
   have been using, which previously worked so
   well, no longer seems to have the same effect.**
   When taste (nursing, bottle feeding) or smell
   (having the child close to you) or touch (cuddling,
   caressing, giving a backrub) no longer predictably

calm, this usually means a child is ready to move into a new developmental phase. Children can look and act restless at this point because they are. They know that something has changed and that they can't settle back into the old way of doing things. But what they don't know yet is what will be their new way of acting in the world or their new way of calming. As a parent, this stage can be very confusing, and our natural instinct is to do more. But really the most important parenting gift is to let children practice more of their own soothing. We have to build trust in the process. No one can learn anything new without some period of adjustment.

If you have been doing 95% of the soothing and calming process at bedtime, you now need to step back a little and only do 75% of the soothing.

When children are sick or overwhelmed

There are other reasons for not soothing well, such as when a child is sick or experiencing a great deal of stress. We can make sense of both these situations by looking at them in relation to the inner sensory pathway.

When we get sick and can sense that something is wrong – think of the fatigue, irritability, or changes in appetite that come just before getting a cold or a flu – it is due to a disturbance in our sense of well-being. If we do not feel well at our core because of infection, injury, toxicity, or exhaustion, we are inwardly out of balance, and connecting to our sense of well-being won't soothe us. It is not enough in that instance to simply disengage from the outside world. What we really need to do is heal. That is why no one soothes easily when they are sick, although resting quietly is important, both immunologically and physiologically, to help us rebalance our inner world.

Most children also have trouble settling and soothing if they are overwhelmed. All of us have trouble inwardly sensing if we are overstimulated by too much engagement with the outer world. Too much external change – such as a move, a separation, the loss of a loved one, or other kinds of unexpected threat or trauma – tips the balance so that outside impressions dominate our consciousness. We instinctively turn our attention to them for our own protection. We don't want to be caught off guard, so our vigilance goes up. Children are not so easily soothed in a stressful situation because they continually redirect their focus back towards vision and the other more outwardly directed senses in order to stay safe.

But if your child is not ill and is not experiencing stress or trauma yet is still not soothing as well as before, it probably means that they are ready to take a step towards more independent self-soothing.

Over-tiredness

There are times when we become so tired that we almost forget how to rest. We are exhausted, yet there is a kind of inner frenzy that insists we must stay on guard – we can't relax too much because someone will need something any minute. This can look like a child who is not happy, no matter what you do ('I want... nothing!'); it can also look like the slightly frantic gaze that comes into a parent's eyes when they have gone months without more than two and a half hours of uninterrupted sleep (something you can observe in many parents of 9-month-old children). Both need help! Both are signs that it is time to open up the developmental process and allow for a new stage in growth. The right thing to do in such a situation may be to pause, stop trying so hard to fix everything, and look behind the behavior to see what is trying to change.

The stutter-step: how a step backward can become a step forward

There is a certain part of parenting that is particularly frustrating, and it is universal. It sneaks up on us at particularly vulnerable times and leads to PBD – Parental Bedtime Despair. This may not be a true clinical diagnosis, but it is certainly a true experience when our carefully practiced sleep technique goes bust. It's usually unexpected and happens when we feel we have finally figured out how to reliably get our children to go to sleep. Having a child who consistently sleeps becomes not just a relief, but a triumph! (Especially after an extended period of sleep deprivation.) But then our soothing technique starts to lose its efficacy and you come down with a bad case of PBD.

There are several variations of this.

A common one in the first months of life goes like this. You've figured out that your child will predictably fall asleep as long as they are resting on your chest. It's a relief to have found an effective soothing method, but then you find that you are stuck. You can't move, literally. As soon as you start to shift your position, the baby wakes up. With an infant that is perhaps not such a big deal – you can put them in a carrier and still get a lot of other things done while they sleep. But as a child gets bigger, having them need to continually lie on your chest the entire time they are asleep becomes cumbersome. Your child grows too big to comfortably carry, but you still desperately need the young one to restfully sleep.

Something similar can occur when your child is older. You can get your child to fall asleep, but as soon as you slip away from their bedside, they wake up in distress. Now the whole soothing process has to start again. This makes bedtime a long process. Sometimes it even becomes a mutual bedtime, where tired parents lie down and also fall asleep. Then they wake some hours later and move to their own bed, although this may only be a temporary respite if their child wakes in the night and comes to get into bed with them.

A third variation is that your child will predictably go to sleep if you gently rub their back, but as soon as you stop stroking, they wake up. You find that, whereas previously you only needed to scratch or rub their back for 1–2 minutes, now you are required to sit there and rub for 10 minutes, 20 minutes, or even more.

In each instance, something that previously worked well starts losing its efficacy and as a parent you feel stuck.

What can you do? Your first thought might be to comfort your child for longer. This is a very common approach to the problem, especially when, as a parent, you are incredibly tired. You give more cuddling, longer backrubs, more songs, an extra story. This is a natural instinct; after all, providing loving comfort and reassurance is a core part of parenting. But so too is helping your child take a step towards more independent self-soothing at the appropriate time. I have spoken with families who stay only with that first approach, continually adding more steps, and end up with a 2-hour bedtime routine. But the very long bedtime actually ends up decreasing the total amount of time a child sleeps.

> Creating space for your child to more actively practice their own self-soothing is usually the best step when a previously successful sleep technique no longer works.

Most of the time *both* the child and the parents feel frustrated that things are not working as well as they used to. The child also wants to find a new and better way to settle. Even though you may fear that making a change will lead to more disruption and less sleep, a good next step is to shift your bedtime routine and do less.

As the parent, you have probably been doing 95% of the soothing process to get your child to go to sleep. Now you need to step back to about 70–80%, which means more of the process is being given to your child as a practice space. This does not mean abandoning your child, but it does mean doing a slightly different parenting job. Your task now is to focus more on providing a good rhythm and a consistent routine for quieting at the end of the day, but it is no longer solely your responsibility to make your child go all the way to sleep.

What does this look like, in practical terms, from the parenting side? It can be simple. In the first few months of life, it means not always nursing or bottle-feeding your child all the way to sleep. Instead, feed them until they are settled and calm but still awake, and then let them try doing the last 10–20% of the calming/sleeping process. Here is the sequence: feed (taste) to a point of satiated, calm wakefulness, then put your child down to fall asleep (not yet completely asleep). If they stir or make a sound, let them be for a few minutes. You have just opened a space for your child to not be solely reliant on taste for soothing. That's a life skill!

If your child is older and you have been lying with them until they fall asleep, once they are tucked in, you can move to a chair, away from the bed, and sing a lullaby or talk about a favorite memory. Close contact (which invariably involves the senses of smell and touch) helped signal that it is time to settle, but now you have opened a space for your child to practice the last part of the self-soothing process. You let them know it's time to get ready – putting on their pajamas, brushing their teeth, reading them a story, giving them a cuddle and tucking them into bed (probably a good two-thirds of the bedtime routine) – and now you create a space for them to do the rest. After a period of adjustment your child will take on this self-soothing practice and move into a new phase.

How long does it usually take to make this shift? There is research showing that, on average, we need about two months to really change a habit. Fortunately, in these windows of developmental change, we have some wind at our back so that things can often move more quickly. Committing to thirty repetitions (one month) of a new soothing pattern is a good baseline. Sometimes parents are surprised to find that it takes only two or three nights to make this shift, even when they have been dreading (for weeks, months, or even years) the disruption that any kind of change might bring. A smooth shift signifies that even though your child demanded more comforting and took longer to soothe, what they actually wanted was more control over the soothing process. And this is what can confuse us.

> If a child is inwardly ready for a shift, but we only offer more of the same outside soothing experiences, we do not help the problem.

A child's growing bedtime distress during these transitional periods comes because they do not feel as reassured, as safe or as oriented as they used to be, despite the increased nursing, rocking, prolonged backrubs, or extended bedtime routines. They are ready to diversify their soothing repertoire. Knowing the sequence of the steps on this inward path (from taste, to smell, to touch) gives us a guide for knowing when and how to make these shifts.

The 'bedtime and 2:00 am' mirroring rule

Whatever sensory experiences a child receives when falling asleep creates the template for how the child wants to be soothed at other times too. That's true whether a child wakes at 2:00 am or feels disoriented in a social situation. If a child has always nursed to fall asleep, then it is only natural that every time they wake in the night they want to nurse (usually when sleep lightens as part of a natural sleep cycle). They will seek taste so that they can be soothed. That will be true every time the child needs to go back to sleep in the night. These 'tasting' feeds have their own character. They are not really a full nurse because they are not about nutrition. Instead, a child latches on, sucks and swallows a few times (just enough to taste sweet milk) and then goes to sleep. At a certain point this pattern becomes exhausting for both the child and their parents, for when a child repeatedly wakes during the night sleep becomes shallower and not as restful. Each time, the child has to wake up, then wake up the parent who provides the milk, before being able to go back to sleep.

Let's look at the same pattern but take taste (nursing) out

of the equation and think of an older child who has their own bed. If bedtime always involves lying down with a child until they are fully asleep, then when they wake in the middle of the night, they are naturally going to seek the smell and touch of their parents in order to go back to sleep. That is a common scenario. Why should we think about this in a new way? Because it means that when we, as parents, even with the best of intentions, create more elaborate and extended bedtime routines, we may just be reinforcing soothing patterns that rely on outer soothing. We hope and pray that a longer, more loving bedtime routine will help our child fall into a deeper sleep so that they will sleep all the way through the night, but we may just be conditioning our child to be dependent on further outer sensory stimulus to settle and sleep. This pattern helps to explain the paradox of why a longer bedtime routine does not necessarily lead to a better night's sleep.

What is the correct timeline for these things? A healthy guideline is that whenever we see our child making significant steps of outer-motor development and exploration, we should look to see if there is a readiness for an accompanying inward shift. Chapter 10 shows the general relationship between the milestones in our outer development and the inward steps that lead to expanded self-awareness and soothing. Here are a couple of common examples of these reciprocal changes.

2–3 months

As an infant's head and neck strength improves, and as the small muscles which move the eyes become more practiced, a child's gaze changes. They can now look up into your face, even if only for a few seconds to begin with. That outward looking is often accompanied by an inner orientation through the sense of smell. For that reason, many babies at this time can be comforted just by the smell of a parent and do not necessarily need to taste in order to soothe.

6-9 months

Sleep commonly becomes disrupted at 6–9 months of age. Napping patterns change, going from perhaps three to two naps per day, and touching, rubbing, bouncing activities do not soothe as well as they used to. This is simultaneously the first phase of real outward exploration, as children go from rolling front to back (around 4 months), to rolling back to front (5 months), to pushing up onto hands and knees, to sitting (6 months), to scooching or 'army crawling' (crawling on their stomach using their elbows), to crawling on their hands and knees (9 months). Not surprisingly, during this time lots of questions come up about sleep. We now know to ask how the process of sleep is going. Is a child stuck somewhere on the 'taste' to 'smell' to 'touch' pathway? More details about working with a stuck sensory process will be explained in Chapter 4. The important learning point is that we need to flip our thinking. We need to stop seeing restlessness as a parenting failure – 'Ugh, my perfect sleep routine is falling apart!' – and instead recognize that restlessness signals a readiness in a child to take the next step in their development.

Quick reminders

★ Your parenting task at bedtime changes over time. The eventual goal is to move towards providing rhythmic, consistent signals that it is time for sleep, without actually having to make your child go to sleep.

★ Be careful about adding more and more soothing experiences from the outside in order to hasten sleep at bedtime, even though that is a very common and generous response. Instead, remember that there are regular developmental windows when what your child most needs is the opportunity to practice their own settling and soothing.

Developmental changes with soothing

★ **2–3 months:** your child can often be soothed with smell (proximity) and may not always need to nurse (taste) to feel reassured.

★ **4–5 months:** when children start true movement exploration (with rolling), this is a good developmental window to start using feeding as a *prelude* to sleep, shifting away from taste as the exclusive way to fall asleep. There is no urgency or mandate for this. Neither should you worry if you have an older child and this didn't happen at that time. But offering space for your child to experiment with a little self-soothing can make future steps toward growth, and associated changes in soothing patterns, easier to navigate.

Tips for improving a stuck soothing process

Closely observe the bedtime routine for your child for at least three nights. Then sit down and take some notes. Consider these questions:

★ How does the bedtime routine flow: is it too short or too long? Where does it tend to get stuck?

★ How would you rate your own level of PBD (Parental Bedtime Despair)? How often do you begin the process already feeling flustered? What part is most frustrating?

★ How much of the bedtime soothing process are you doing? What percentage?

★ Are the steps for going to bed predictable and consistent or is it a free-for-all that changes all the time? Does your child know when it is time to shift from receiving outside soothing to practicing more inward quieting and self-orientation?

★ Are there particular steps in the process where you can see your child visibly relax? Are they connected to particular sensory experiences, such as taste, smell or touch?

These observations will help provide the building blocks for creating a new bedtime routine. We will explore these more in the next chapter.

4. FINDING BALANCE FROM AGE 1 ONWARD

Consciousness, and the need for soothing, takes another big leap forward at around 1 year of age. This is the time when most children begin to pull up to a standing position. A child's relationship to the world changes with that upright position, not just because it is a different view but because the foundations for greater independence are being built. Children first 'cruise' while holding onto a piece of furniture. Then, when they are ready, they adventure out with teetering steps. Between 12 and 15–18 months of age, cruising becomes toddling, which becomes steady walking (see Chapter 10, which charts these gross-motor and fine-motor milestones). Another core reason why a toddler's awareness changes is because the sense of balance wakes up. The relationship of self and the outside world intensifies as a child actively explores their sense of balance. Through standing and walking, they find a new level of independent awareness.

Balance is different from taste, smell and touch because it doesn't rely on any outside influence. In fact, you cannot guide another person's sense of balance from the outside;

it is based on a special kind of self-perception. Rocking a child in your arms or pushing them on a swing does, of course, stimulate a child's vestibular organs in the inner ear, but the self-orienting aspect must be individually learned and practiced. Once a child learns to pull themselves up to a standing position, the swinging or rocking motions provided by an adult become only a very small part of any child's experience of balance. Awareness of balance comes through perceiving the position of one's body in relationship to the outside environment. Am I steady? Am I tipping over? Where is the middle?

Balance provides a more dynamic sense of self than any of the previous sense experiences. It simultaneously helps us venture out more independently and anchors us more deeply in our own experience. Rudolf Steiner described the sense of balance in this way:

> If we press still further into our interior, we come upon a sense which is usually no longer mentioned, as least not often. It is a sense by which we differentiate between our standing up or lying down, and through which we perceive when we are standing on our own two feet, that we are in a state of balance. This experience of equilibrium is transmitted by the sense of balance. There, we penetrate completely into our interior; we perceive the relationship of our own inner being to the world outside, within which we experience ourselves in a state of equilibrium. We perceive this, however, entirely within our inner being.[1]

Let's place the sense of balance in our inner sensory pathway:

Vision > Taste > Smell >
Touch > **Balance** >>> Well-Being

After 1 year of age, a child's possibilities for soothing diversify. Children do indeed get a little restless at this time because they are reorienting. The other senses we have already discussed are also shifting around this one-year mark.

Taste and nursing

The self-soothing role of taste sees a remarkable shift in this 12–15-month period. Children by this time have enough front teeth to bite food and some accompanying molars to chew. They can take in a broader variety of foods. Digestive activity – which is, of course, different from crawling or walking but shares similar developmental patterns because it is another way to interact with the outside world – matures enough so that children are usually able to eat a broad diet. There still needs to be awareness of texture (avoiding nuts, hard chips, chunks of meat), but specially prepared baby foods are no longer necessary. Put another way: parents no longer need to be so involved in every aspect of the nutritive process by either exclusively providing nutrition from their own body (producing milk) or continually selecting and preparing specific types and consistencies of food (such as cooking and pureeing vegetables). A 12–15-month-old child has greater capacities and can take on more of the digesting and nourishing process. Experiences of taste also evolve as food is eaten rhythmically at meals, and in such a way that taste is no longer so directly linked to the soothing/sleeping process. More times than not, eating is no longer followed by sleep. This is quite different from the newborn baby who routinely fell asleep after every nurse or bottle. We are entering into a different developmental stage.

There is a natural cohort of children who become much less interested in nursing at around 12–15 months. Given the shift in the sense of taste, this is understandable. The orientation of these children is changing. They do not easily settle down to nurse at the breast or bottle and are instead more interested in everything else that is happening around them. This outer behavioral shift reflects an evolving inner soothing pathway: children are now additionally able to self-orient through smell, touch, and balance. This means that the developmental window when children are learning to stand, to balance and to walk, provides a natural window for many children to wean from breast or bottle. This does not mean that every child must wean during this time. It also does not mean that there should be negative judgments if a child nurses for a shorter or longer period than 12–15 months. What it does offer is an invitation to look with an open mind at your own child and see how their developmental anchors are evolving.

Some families have shared with me that they did see this window but because they didn't understand or pay attention to it, they encouraged their child to continue breastfeeding. What happens for some children is that the soothing and sleeping process then becomes much more of a push-and-pull battle. Why? Because on the one hand they continue to rely strongly on an outward source for soothing, yet on the other they are no longer fully soothed by this tasting process. They need more and frequent outer soothing but are not satisfied with it. That kind of extended developmental stutter-step cannot always be easily anticipated. Sometimes it just happens – but when you find yourself in the middle of a prolonged push-and-pull battle, the most helpful support often is to help your child find more independent practices for self-soothing.

For a certain group of children I have met in my medical practice, the persistent linkage of taste and soothing (nursing beyond 2–3, or even 4 years) has observably complicated their ability to self-soothe. They are conflicted. They have become independent in so many aspects of life, yet predictably exhibit strong insecurity in social situations when they are away from their outer anchor, their parent. They become stuck, exhibiting increasing anxiety even as both child and parent fear making any kind of shift. In truth, making a shift does not mean that as parents we love our children any less. If we can see the stutter-step happening, it's a sign that they are ready for us to love and guide them in a different way, and that they are actually ready to become more active participants in their own soothing and calming.

Other developmental changes also come with the shift towards more independent capacities for movement at

12–18 months. The changes are not just about taste. Coming into awareness of the sense of balance also brings expanded self-awareness on social and emotional levels.

Falling down and running away

Our sense of balance tells us about the position of our body in relation to our environment, whether we are jumping or running away, standing up or lying down. All of these perceptions are made possible by the three semi-circular canals in the inner ear, the core organs of our vestibular system. But beyond the purely mechanical sensing of position and orientation, an awakening sense of balance brings with it a broader awareness of how we relate to our environment.

Spatial awareness of the relationship between one's body and the environment helps maintain uprightness, which is anything but static. Standing upright requires that we continuously sense and adjust the relationship between our body and the outside – think of balancing on one foot, for example, or walking on a balance beam. A toddler's new-found awareness of balance brings the first glimmers of there being a 'self' and a separate 'environment'. It's a new sensation and toddlers want to experience it over and over again. They stand and fall and stand and fall, then they step and fall and so on. Repetition brings practiced awareness.

The experience of relating a separate self to its environment also plays out on an emotional and social level through the experience of contrasts. Up until now a child's sense of well-being has been primarily dictated by their strong connection to parents and caregivers. Their world has basically been one big whole. When children start to feel that they have a self within and a world outside, they realize that they are separate, and they feel the strong need to practice connection and separation – another kind of equilibrium.

The three semi-circular canals in our inner ear help us to sense contrasting qualities and to accurately sense if we are moving up or down, leaning to the left or to the right, tipping forward or backward. The physical structures for this awareness have, of course, been present from birth, but as children learn to walk, they work with that balance input in a new way. The child notices, more and more: 'How do I feel?'

That capacity for contrasting qualities shows itself emotionally through alternating states of excitement and fear, fatigue and energy, sympathy and antipathy. Moving between connection and isolation allows independent impulses to bubble up. Suddenly the wishes of a child stop corresponding to the plans of the adults.

Have you ever needed to chase a toddler down, because they got going with their independent mobility and ran away from you? That can be a great game, one that they want to practice over and over, even if you are telling them they should stop. That is part of the practice of feeling themselves in relationship to the outside world. Over and over children work to strengthen their capacity for feeling: 'I have my own impulse! I can feel what I want to do, even if (perhaps especially if) it is different from what you are telling me to do!'

Escaping toddlers
and repeated refusals

By 18 months of age the sense of balance reaches a new level of maturity. Most children can walk independently and climb stairs while holding someone's hand. Their strengthened sense of balance allows them to squat down to pick up an object and then stand up again without falling over. All of this takes a lot of sensing and orientation.

Social and emotional changes also occur around this time. Children begin to say 'No!' a lot. This is because they sense that there is a 'self' and an 'other', which allows for an alternating dynamic of connection (sympathy) and separation (antipathy). These routine refusals, infamously known as the 'Terrible Twos', follow soon after the toddler escape routines, when children experiment with their physical independence by running away.

One reason why this shift is so interesting to observe is that even when a child says 'No', much of their behavior remains imitative. After refusing a bite of food they will often, in the very next moment, open their mouth and then happily chew and swallow. Such strong bouts of refusal quickly pass. Swings of antipathetic refusal and sympathetic cooperation shift from moment to moment. A child who won't do anything you ask them to, and then gets upset and has a tantrum one moment, often needs hugs and reassurance that everything is fine the next. 18–24-month-old children seek ways to exercise their own impulses, but they are still too little and too dependent to really sustain them. Saying 'No' is one of the main ways that children try out repetitive experiences of separation and connection. It is important to remember that these refusals are an experiment in balance. They are not deep moral judgments, nor are they true expressions of what a child actually likes or needs. They are a developmental stage of practicing balance.

How do you navigate these kinds of negotiations?

Remember: they aren't really negotiations; they're practice for sensing self and surroundings. Bringing in more intellectual methods of questioning and reasoning won't work at this age. We might be tempted to ask questions, thinking it will make this stage easier. In the adult world, checking to see if someone is ready to cooperate is generally the best way to go, but that kind of discussion is developmentally out of place for a 2-year-old. Negotiating with a child who is vigorously practicing experiences of separation is a quick way to either create more conflict or teach your child to start ignoring what you say. For example, if it is time to go and you ask a 2-year-old whether they are ready to put on their shoes and the child says 'No!' you have a potential battle looming. Either you are going to have to override your child's will or you are going to leave with a shoeless child. Other times it's not a battle, but instead feels more like a waste of time. You ask them if they're ready to put on their shoes and they say 'No!', but when you ask them if they'd rather not wear any shoes they again say 'No!' Then you realize that the whole conversation has really just been a sense-of-balance practice session.

Like it or not, the Terrible Twos is a good age for practicing your own parental equilibrium. Usually that means focusing on the task at hand and not being too dismayed with escaping toddlers or repeated refusals. A good practice for when it does feel important to ask your child a question is to pose a question where both answers are going to be the right answer: 'Should we put the shoe on this foot first or on this foot first?' Avoiding yes/no questions can be hugely helpful for getting through those times when refusal is not a good option.

This is a lesson I've learned well as a physician. Small children are understandably nervous about being examined by a strange adult. This is especially true if they are meeting you for the first time, or if they don't feel well. The whole interaction can be scary, uncomfortable and threatening. For example, if a child is being brought in for fever, restlessness, and irritability ten days into a cold, then I have to look in the ears to know what is going on. Is an ear infection causing all the discomfort? In that moment, asking if it's OK to look in the child's ears and being told 'No' makes for a very unhappy visit! It works much better to instead ask a question to which all answers are correct.

'Which ear should we look in first?'

Or alternatively: 'Where is your ear?' and 'How many ears do you have?'

These kinds of questions leave space for a response without immediately setting up a power struggle.

What does all of this opposition bring? What does a child gain by saying 'No' so many times? The answer is an *enhanced sense of self.*

> It is challenging to parent a child who repeatedly rejects everything, but that balancing capacity for feeling what is 'me' and what is 'not-me' provides a necessary ingredient of resilience.

This allows for a more continuous experience of self, and developing a stronger sense of self provides a counterweight to the demands of the outside world. That inner anchoring protects us from being bowled over by all the unpredictable events that happen around us.

Exercising the dynamics of self/not-self happens repeatedly over the course of a lifetime; we do not work with it just once. The sense of balance is revisited during early adolescence, when waves of sympathy and antipathy once more strongly influence the experience of self and environment. There is a certain developmental mirroring between 18–30 months and 12–14 years of age.

The 2–3-year-old's practice of balance builds the foundation for later capacities of differentiation as they learn to connect and disconnect from other people. It is largely an instinctual process, not necessarily planned, strategic or rational. Puberty brings another round of practice with the sense of balance, only now it plays out on primarily a social level. Whereas at around the age of 2 a child practices rejection mainly as a way of feeling and defining *themselves*, 12–14-year-olds are practicing the dynamic of self and *other*. Emotions swing strongly, with newfound experiences of love and isolation, of enthusiasm and apathy. Rejection of childish things alternates with fear about becoming a teenager and eventually an adult. These older adolescent swings are not easy, but they are vital for continuing to shape the sense of self.

These experiences build on each other. In other words, navigating the shifting social currents of early adolescence will be easier when a child has been able to thoroughly engage with the sense of balance through toddling, walking, and rejecting, between the ages of 2 and 3 years (you can read more about the pairing of different developmental thresholds in Chapter 10).

Finding a healthy sense of balance comes not through instruction, but through practice. As has been mentioned, the sense of balance is an orienting process that cannot be managed from the outside, unlike taste, smell, and touch. That means it will be a little messy. Children do not find their uprightness without first tipping and leaning many different times.

Quick reminders

★ When you see your child pulling to a stand or beginning to walk, a new phase of development and self-awareness is beginning. Through practicing and experiencing the sense of balance, your child's whole awareness of self and environment is beginning to change.

★ Between 12 and 18 months, the role of taste changes. This is a vital time to support other, additional sensory pathways for soothing, and a big way to do this is to allow space for your child to practice and branch into those other senses, particularly touch and balance.

★ Strengthening and developing the sense of balance requires a kind of practice that cannot be coached from the outside. We each must develop our *own* sense of balance. Children need to be allowed space to practice this balancing activity, otherwise they may stay stuck in younger sensory patterns for all their calming and soothing needs.

5. RHYTHMS AND ROUTINES FROM AGE 1 ONWARD

Becoming less dependent on the outside environment means that children can gain more connection to their own physiological needs. We can see this quite clearly if we go back to the example of food and the way that children, from around 1–3 years of age, become able to nourish themselves in new ways. During this time, children gain more teeth and develop more robust digestive activity, as well as a broader palate. They control more of the eating process: biting, chewing, swallowing, and digesting, first with finger foods then with a spoon, cup, and fork.

Inwardly, their digestive capacity is also making great strides. Children at this age start to know when they are hungry. They seek regular snacks. They don't just wait for food to be brought to them; they can now actively sense they need it and better communicate their needs. They want to participate more in the process. One of the best ways to strengthen the inward aspects of digestion is for food to come at predictable times. Young children love to know when they are going to eat! Not in an intellectual way, as when they are told that food is coming, but rather having predictable schedules for both taking in food and then having the time to digest.

This might seem counter-intuitive, because this is also the time when children are actively refusing all kinds of things, but building consistent meal and snack times does foster inner balance. If a 2-year-old learns that there will be lunch at 12:15 pm every day and this becomes a consistent rhythm, then at 12:05 pm their stomach acid will start to increase and their whole digestive activity will ramp up. A child quickly learns to (physiologically) anticipate a meal, and the ability to inwardly prepare means that they will break down the food and absorb it in a more complete way. Children are most fully nourished when they eat and digest with a predictable rhythm.

In much the same way, consistent nap and bedtimes are not only possible, but also quite powerful. If bedtime is consistently at 7:00 pm (yes, 7:00 pm, which is actually a very healthy bedtime for children from 12–24 months, or even earlier – more about that on page 117), then a child will begin to feel sleepy at around 6:40 pm. Children's physiological systems learn to know these rhythms and like these rhythms. The quieter, often underappreciated parts of our life-sustaining physiology love it when they can successfully anticipate, participate, and then inwardly work through what has been taken in.

Now, if lunch is at 11:30 am one day, 1:15 pm the next and 12:30 pm the third day, there is no way for a consistent, inner physiological rhythm to be established. In the same way, if the timing for going to sleep is different every night, waiting to see when our child seems tired, or when we as parents are tired, we rob our child of the needed practice for building inner, physiological 'balance'. The balance here is not so much between sympathy and antipathy, or connection and independence, it is now the balance between eating and digesting, between engaging and resting. Many sleep challenges at this age are related to children being overly tired or being unable to create an inner rhythm.

How consistent does everything have to be to in order to build and maintain these inner rhythms? This will vary from child to child, but a good rule of thumb is that if things are consistent six days out of seven, then rhythms will generally be maintained. This means a belated bedtime on the weekend or a skipped snack or mealtime on a hectic weekday will be fine, but multiple late nights or repeatedly changing sleep or meal rhythms (even between weekdays and weekends) will be hard on a child.

Just as physical balancing (standing, walking, running) and social balancing ('No!') lay the foundation for the emotional balancing of adolescent development, so do rhythmic experiences of sleeping and eating lay the foundation for overall self-regulation. This rhythmic encouragement of a child's physiology to better engage with daily activities helps them create a stronger connection to their own well-being. They begin to sense more clearly 'What do I need?' and 'How do I feel?'

Bedtime rhythms and routines

Sleep rhythms are characteristically quite up and down and require flexibility. It can feel like every time a sleep routine becomes settled and you start to relax, it suddenly stops working. This happens most commonly when a child is over-tired or has just taken a new step towards greater, outer awareness (see Chapter 3, page 43). Moving to a new home, travel, new siblings, illnesses and overscheduling all act as disruptors. Repeatedly working to create predictable, dependable eating and sleeping rituals helps.

Re-establishing consistency is of course particularly difficult when everyone is tired. Here is an observation that, while it may seem a little counter-intuitive, can help. The number of parenting activities that happen in and around a child's bed at this time can be simplified. In other words, if a child is having trouble falling asleep in their bed, do less in and around the bed. Our instincts might tell us something quite different, namely that if our child is struggling to relax and fall asleep, the best thing to do is to make sure they feel extra calm and secure in bed.

> The best way to make bed feel like a safe place for resting is to make it a place that is only for rest.

We can take a cue from adult sleep hygiene. If, as an adult, you are having trouble falling asleep, then a standard recommendation is to limit your bed to two activities: sleep and intimacy. Your bed should not be a place for watching TV, catching up on emails, eating, or reading for hours at a time. This recommendation works because limiting your activities sends a message to your mind (and your physiological systems) that your bed is a place for rest. A similar kind of simplification also helps children at the toddler stage.

Here is how you can make that shift.

As children become more mobile and their soothing/sleeping process shifts away from a reliance on taste, relocate most of the bedtime activities out of the bedroom and into a common social space, like a sofa in the living room. That now becomes the place where, after bathing, changing into pajamas, and brushing teeth, a cozy corner can be created for reading stories, singing songs, snuggling, and sharing. These are all important ways for marking the end of the day and transitioning towards sleep, so we don't want to get rid of them. But just as a child's awareness is shifting at this age, so too can the *parenting goals* around sleep evolve and begin to change. It's already been said, but it bears repeating, especially in this context: your parenting task should move away from doing a whole variety of things until your child falls asleep.

> Build a bedtime routine that consistently signals the end of the day so that your child's nervous system can start to settle and quiet down.

Once you have had this calming period together in a communal space, move to your child's bedroom. This transition – marked by a change of place at a specific moment – creates a signal that it is time for your child to rest quietly and practice falling asleep. The main time for parental interaction has finished.

Why should you make this change in your routine? Let's consider what happens when most or all of the bedtime routine happens in the bed.

If the usual pattern is for your child to climb into bed and then hear several bedtime stories, when does that story time end? Is it after two stories, after three, after eight? It's the same with cuddling and talking. When does that finish? One hug, two hugs, five hugs? Stories, cuddling, talking, and backrubs are all wonderful parts of loving and nurturing your child, and you absolutely want to provide them, but when those bedtime activities shift to a more social space outside of the bedroom, then you are able to give more consistent signals to your child about when they need to practice more independent soothing. Remember the connection described at the beginning of the book about observing a link between children who become agitated or disruptive in social situations and who also struggle with falling asleep at night (see page 11)? That connection exists because those are frequently children who have not had the opportunity to really practice their own skills for calming and self-soothing. When we change the bedtime routine in this way, it helps to build a clear and consistent rhythm, with a time and place for interaction (the sofa) and a time and place for rest (the child's bed).

Now let's take a moment to consider what can go wrong with this plan.

The first, most likely challenge will be protest from your child. This is going to be a new routine and it will naturally bring some disorientation. The whole family may be fearful about making a change, especially if sleep is already a struggle and everyone is tired. Some parents and caregivers feel reluctant to make a change because with their current bedtime routine, even if they have to spend a long time with their child, they do eventually go to sleep. What will happen if you make this kind of shift? It's very possible that your child will appear more restless, moving around in bed, rolling over, stretching, and rubbing as if trying to find a comfortable position. This may feel like a step backwards, but let's explore those behaviors a little bit.

Firstly, there will naturally be a gap when space is opened up for your child to more actively practice quieting down. That sounds like an oxymoron – actively quieting – but that is our goal and we shouldn't be afraid of it. The work of self-orientation and self-soothing will help to build a life skill; it just needs repetition. Most children start settling into this new arrangement after just a few days or a week, even if they complain loudly at the beginning. Don't give up on the shift too soon; every one of us, child or adult, needs about a month before a new pattern starts to feel normal. It is essential to leave a bit of wiggle room for wiggling!

Secondly, as a child grows, more pathways for soothing become available (taste, smell, touch, balance). The further they proceed along the sensory pathway, the more your child will have to independently engage with their own sense activities. It should come as no surprise to find that a child who is seeking more independent ways to calm will engage their senses of touch and balance.

What about a child who rolls over repeatedly or rocks to go to sleep?

Those are methods for harnessing the sense of balance. Think for a moment about your own sleep patterns. Are you out as soon as your head hits the pillow? Or do you need to shift and tuck your pillows just right? Do you start on your stomach and then roll on to your back before finally ending up on your side? These soothing patterns are not unique to childhood. We make use of them all the time. What could be labeled as agitated or restless behavior may in truth be a way for practicing self-soothing and self-orienting through the senses of touch and balance.

> When a child wriggles, shifts position, or rubs while lying in their bed they are engaging with their own sensing activity to experience boundaries and to orient themselves through the sense of touch.

Allow some space for your child to try these out before you intervene. Giving your child space to practice these sensing pathways at bedtime will also help them to more easily settle themselves if they wake in the middle of the night. This will make it easier for them to eventually sleep all the way through.

A question that often comes into this discussion is: what happens if you move story time, sharing, hugging and cuddling to the parents' bed? While that will still help designate your child's own bed as a place more associated with quiet rest, it shifts the main social space to the parents' bed. That might work fine at bedtime, as it still includes the aspect of a place-and-time transition into your child's bedroom, but it tends to encourage more middle-of-the-night visits back to the parents' bed. The best pattern is really one that makes all the beds in the house places for sleeping, and which designates the living room (or whatever other space you choose) as the social space where everyone will gather again in the morning to be together.

An example bedtime routine

1. Pajamas: either putting them on or collecting them to put on after a bath. This marks the first important step in the transition towards bedtime, indicating that daytime clothes and activities are no longer needed and are finished.

2. Bathing: face washing, toothbrushing, and going to the bathroom.

3. Calming activities: gather in an inviting, quiet social space (no TV, no music) for talking, stories, and cuddling. This is also helpful if you are trying to get multiple children to bed in multiple bedrooms, as then there isn't the need for an elaborate bedtime routine in each child's bedroom.

4. Transition to the bedroom: when those bedtime activities have finished, move to the bedroom and into bed. This transition can be a challenging step, but having a silly song to sing about going to bed, or offering a ride on a parents' backs, or having the child stand on your feet and grab on to your legs to get a 'foot ride' into their bedroom, can all be great helpers. Additional bathroom stops or desperately needed drinks of water often seem to sneak in at this stage, but try not to let them interrupt the flow.

5. Bed: when your child is in bed, decide on one or two final, simple, predictable activities – a verse, a poem, a prayer, or a lullaby are all good choices. It's good if it's something that your child can also begin to say or sing. In time, your child can invoke those words or tunes as a way to calm themselves.

How long should these activities be? Just a couple of minutes. Repeated personal and professional experience shows that when this kind of element consistently comes at the end of bedtime, a child will frequently yawn before the verse or song is done. Remember, you are not expecting your child to fall asleep during such a short verse or song. The verse or song (or yawn) provides a meaningful step towards rest.

One key reason for suggesting this kind of shorter soothing activity in the bedroom is that if you do need to go back in to help settle and calm your child after 10 or 15 minutes, you can do the same bit of ritual – a song, a verse, a hug – but now in an even more abbreviated form. If it comes with a consistent message that social time is over and you will only be giving short, repeated interaction or reassurance, then episodes of bedtime tug of war lessen. If you find you need to go back into the bedroom multiple times, try doing an ever more abbreviated tucking in. If your child is still not settling and you have done it three or four times, then get them up for a while and try taking them back to their bed later, when they seem sleepy. If it feels like a failure, start again the next evening. With repetition, the new bedtime routine will become the new normal. Look at your calendar and mark out the days. To fully set a new pattern often takes 4–6 weeks, though some children settle into a new pattern after just a couple of nights.

Healthy balance is not a static state. It comes from maintaining a flexible equilibrium between inside and outside: from rhythmically eating and digesting to practicing waking and sleeping. Feeling different kinds of connection and separation not only helps a child experience more independence, but it also builds greater capacities for navigating the outside world's many impressions and demands. By developing and refining the sense of balance, children create and claim an inner world, a place they can retreat to and regroup. Each child's learning to stand and walk, to rhythmically eat and digest, and to know when it is time to rest, forms the foundation for greater resilience in a busy world.

Tips for choosing bedtime verses

There is complete freedom when choosing a bedtime verse, poem, or lullaby. Lullabies exist in every culture and language, for the need to quiet and calm children is universal. Choose something that reflects your own experience and heritage (I still get a little dreamy when I sing the lullabies sung to me as a child) or discover something completely new.

Find something that you can sing or speak with your child, which is much better than purchasing a recording. Recordings may be beautiful, but they remain an outside experience and do not have the same quality as your voice. Helping your child learn to sing or speak something together will, in time, help them make this end-of-the-day practice their own. Then your child can call it up, whenever needed, wherever they are, without being dependent on an outside sensory experience.

A personal favorite of my own children was the poem 'Wynken, Blynken and Nod' by Eugene Field. You can easily find the full text through an internet search. It shares lovely imagery, though it is a long poem (which might be fine for a 2- or 3-year-old but is probably too much for an older child). In general, just take the amount of a poem or verse that feels manageable and helpful.

Quick reminders

★ Consistent rhythms for mealtimes and bedtime allow a child to feel what is coming. That helps them eat better and sleep better (and in time will reduce arguing and negotiating around these everyday activities).

★ Building a bedtime routine, with consistent steps, clearly marks when it is the end of the day, and signals that now it is time to rest.

★ The toddler to 2-year-old phase is a good time to open space for 'active quieting'. Let your child roll, move, fuss a little before you intervene. Leave space for your child to explore and find their own self-soothing patterns.

Questions to consider

Look back at the notes you took at the end of Chapter 2. What have you learned? Perhaps it would be useful to consider a few more things:

★ What works well about the way you are helping your child go to bed?

★ Where do you see your child practicing the sense of balance?

★ Are there any changes you would like to make in terms of the sequence or different components of bedtime?

★ Write a short parenting 'job description', focusing on the question: what is my role at bedtime?

6. WHEN OLDER CHILDREN STRUGGLE TO SLEEP AND SETTLE

Sleep rhythms typically need to be adjusted several times. Not everything magically unfolds during the toddler stage. What happens if your 4-year-old child who is battling bedtime frequently wakes in the middle of the night and still requires lots of outside calming and reassurance? What if your 8-year-old cannot fall asleep without a parent present? The answer is that the different sensing capacities along this inward pathway still need to be nurtured and practiced. The main difference is that an older child is usually ready to take bigger steps along that pathway.

How and when a child makes a shift towards settling more independently is never written in stone; there are, or course, as many variations as there are children. There is a danger that as soon as we define any kind of 'typical' range, we are labeling a whole group of children who do not fit that pattern as 'abnormal'. That is not the intention. The timing can be quite individual; the most important aspect is the progression.

If your child is stuck on taste

If your child is having a hard time moving away from taste as the primary sense experience for soothing (they are still nursing or bottle feeding) and won't let that go, then you can encourage a shift by bringing more experiences of smell. Smell is the next sense on the inner pathway:

Vision > Taste **> Smell** > Touch >
Balance > Movement >>> Well-being

Having a beloved blanket or stuffed animal is one way to reassure a child through the sense of smell. If you recognize that your child needs to practice settling without taste, try moving a pillowcase that has been on a parent's pillow for several days to the child's pillow. That will bring some familiar smell. Another option is to introduce a pleasant smell into your bedtime routine, a smell that will stay with your child without you needing to be physically present for the whole time they are falling asleep. There are safe, natural creams and body oils – with ingredients like rose, lavender, or chamomile – that are naturally calming. Through repeating the same familiar smell and incorporating it into a rhythmic bedtime routine (see Chapter 5, page 69), your child will soon learn to associate a particular smell with the quieting process.

Creams, body oils, or ointments are usually best incorporated as one of the last steps when tucking your child into bed, though they can be given earlier as part of the preparation for story time (perhaps when brushing teeth or putting on pajamas). The pleasant smell gently signals that the day is coming to an end and that it is time for your child's nervous system to shift into a more relaxed and regenerative mode. It's worth emphasizing that this is meant to support and simplify the settling process – don't let it become a complex extension of the bedtime routine. Children older than 3 years can usually apply a cream or ointment themselves by rubbing some on their chest. In this way they are also learning to mark the transition themselves: 'This is my task; I know how to do it.' Rubbing on a small amount of cream or oil also brings a self-engendered experience of touch. Even the use of a gentle, natural soap for face-washing can have the same effect.

These kinds of consistent smell experiences offer a next sensory 'foothold' for a child on this inner pathway once taste experiences have expanded and are no longer so closely linked to the soothing process.

We all experience the signaling activity of smells. Any smell that you associate with your own bedtime preparation – a toothpaste, a lotion, even the detergent smell of your sheets – has a similar, subtle effect.

If your child is stuck on touch

Touch is another very common place to become stuck on the pathway of self-soothing. With smaller children this might show itself through a pattern of you needing to carry or hold them until they fall asleep, then finding that they stir as soon as you try to move them or set them down (of course, your special comforting smell is there too). A related pattern for an older child might be when they want you to lie next to them while they fall asleep, or they want you to give them a back-rub or they want to stroke your arm until they fall asleep. The consistent pattern is that touch needs to be there for a child to fully relax.

The fact that these are all common, loving ways for us to show affection adds a level of nuance. We should indeed cradle and calm and reassure children through the sense of touch, and we should not be afraid to show our care through touch. But when does it become too much?

An important sign that your child might be stuck on this particular sense is when calming touch needs to be given for longer and longer periods and instead of reassuring them it becomes part of a power struggle. You sense that while one part of your child's body is slowly relaxing, there is also a vigilant 'sonar' activity sending out little *pings* to verify that you, the parent, haven't gone away. *Ping! Ping! Ping!*

When a child tries on one level to relax into sleep, yet simultaneously works to keep their touch antennae wide open to make sure their parent hasn't left, this creates conflict. It produces a metaphorical pressure on both 'brake' (sleeping) and 'gas pedal' (active sensing) at the same time. This conflicted process can then get locked into a repeated confrontation, with both the parents and child worried about the coming ordeal, even before they get to bed.

When sleep patterns become locked into this kind of conflicted, worried anticipation, the most helpful step is to bring a kind of breathing rhythm into the process.

How do we do this? By offering deep, slow, reassuring touch and then allowing a pause for the experience to settle. Touch first comes from the outside, slow and confident, but with enough insistence that a child can really feel themselves, as opposed to them focusing on maintaining contact with the outside.

We've already heard about the special quality of touch and that when we touch objects what we actually perceive is ourselves (see page 31). Children stuck on touch long for continued touch as a way to reinforce a sense of boundary between inside and outside. We can foster the next step on the inner sensory pathway by encouraging children to really, physically, feel themselves through deep touch.

We could compare this to when a fly lands on the back of your neck. Usually, it is an uncomfortable sensation because you can feel some encounter with the outside world, but not feel it enough to know where your boundary actually lies. Typically, we react by swatting at the fly (in order to get the sensation to go away), then we scratch or slap or rub the area. Why do we scratch, slap, and rub? In order to have a strong enough touch experience that we can sense ourselves fully, feel a clear boundary between our self and the outside world.

For the purposes of promoting a smoother and happier bedtime, here is a description of what in my practice has been fondly named the 'Toothpaste Treatment'. It has proven valuable with hundreds, if not thousands of children at this point, although there is no age limit for it. I've taught it to groups of doctors who have even found it helpful in calming and reassuring much older adults living in nursing homes. We can always use help feeling our boundary with the outside world to relax more into our inner world.

Toothpaste Treatment

All children love stories, so this touch exercise has a story to go along with it. This is how it is usually told to young children in the medical office:

> Sometimes when I am getting ready for bed and I am already in my pajamas, I go to brush my teeth and find that the toothpaste tube is almost empty! Now I really don't want to go to the store and get a new tube of toothpaste because I am already in my pajamas, so what do I do?

Answers at this point vary, with a surprising range of suggestions. Many children quickly understand, however, that you have to squeeze the tube in order to get the last little bits of toothpaste out.

> Yes, I need to get some last toothpaste out. So what I do is I take the tube of toothpaste and, starting at the end, I slowly squeeze all the way along the tube so that I can get enough toothpaste out to brush my teeth. Now, what if we pretend that your arm is a tube of toothpaste, and we squeeze it and see if we can get any toothpaste to come out of the tips of your fingers?

Most young children are a little bit curious by this point, so they willingly offer an arm. If a child is older, perhaps finishing kindergarten or elementary school age, then I often add an introduction along the lines of:

> There is a really nice way to make your arm feel relaxed and to help you calm down. I would like to show it to you. It's called the Toothpaste Treatment and if you were a lot younger then I would tell you the story behind the name (even though I know you are probably too big for a story like this). Here is the story I tell: 'Sometimes when I am getting ready for bed, and I am already in my pajamas...'

The imagination is still important for an older child and helps them relax into feeling the slow, deep pressure. Here's the technique:

1. Start towards the top of one of the upper arms and, using both of your hands, squeeze the arm slowly, the same way that a blood pressure cuff squeezes. Make sure you apply touch all the way around the arm, from all sides. You can put your thumbs right next to each other, pointing up towards the shoulder, then wrap your palms and fingers around, overlapping your fingers if your hands are big enough to go all the way around (Figure 6.1).

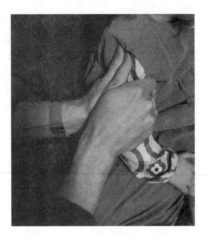

Figure 6.1

2. Squeeze slowly and firmly, slower than might be your first instinct, and hold it. Usually squeezing and holding for 6–8 seconds is a good amount of time.

3. Then move down the arm and repeat the squeezing. Repeat this until you have gone all the way down the arm. Avoid squeezing right over the elbow joint, just above and below is sufficient, and stop when you get to the wrist. The total number of squeezes depends on the relative size of your hands to the size of your child's arm: 4–6 squeezes is probably enough.

4. If you are pushing in equally from all sides, you can use a good amount of strength and pressure. If the pressure is too light or too fast, it will feel unsettling (think of the fly crawling on your neck).

5. When you get to the hand, squeeze that too, but from the front and back. You can place your child's hand between your palms and squeeze (kind of like a waffle iron). Give consistent, deep, gentle pressure (Figure 6.2).

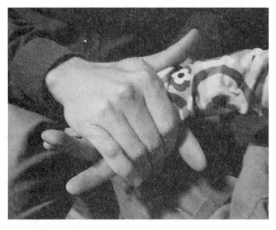

Figure 6.2

6. Then, taking your index finger and thumb, start at the base of each finger and thumb and slowly pull along the top and bottom of the finger, out towards the fingertip (you can even invite your child to look to see if there is any toothpaste coming out!). This should again be slow, consistent, and firm. The pressure is mainly directed inwards on the finger or thumb, with only a very mild motion pulling outward on it (Figure 6.3).

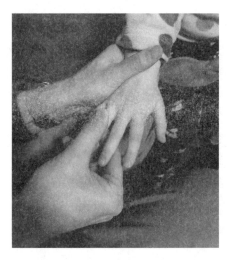

Figure 6.3

★ If your child seems uncomfortable at any point, stop. This should never hurt or be uncomfortable; this needs to be a nurturing experience. Don't apply pressure to any place that is swollen, tender, or injured. If your child seems initially unsure, focus most on giving steady, deep touch and make sure there is time for it to settle, settle, settle.

★ If you are doing it in a slow, gentle way, many children will spontaneously offer you their second arm as you complete the first. Usually, their breathing also becomes slower and more relaxed. That is a sign that your child is really being nourished by your touch.

★ On multiple occasions, after slowly and gently giving this treatment to children on both their arms, and sometimes on their legs as well, parents have commented that their child looks calmer than they have ever seen them. That's a clear sign that the child needs a lot more practice at feeling this deeper connection to self in a safe, unrushed way.

★ If a child feels threatened by the process, it won't work. A child can't relax into feeling that deeper sense of self if they are unsure or guarded about what you are doing. Pushing on tense or flexed muscles is much more likely to feel uncomfortable.

The Toothpaste Treatment is usually best incorporated into your bedtime routine when you are still together in a common social space, sharing stories, snuggling, or talking. This offering of deep touch should have a beginning and an end and not be too long, perhaps doing one or two arms one evening (3–5 minutes), one or two legs the next evening (3–5 minutes). The same technique can be used for the legs, except now you start at the mid-thigh and work down to the feet and toes.

After a while, just a little bit of this gentle, reassuring pressure will help center your child. While out at a social gathering, or before being dropped off in a kindergarten classroom, a slow squeeze of the shoulders or a long, leaning hug can have the same kind of centering effect. Children learn that they gain something valuable through this experience of touch, with some proactively requesting the Toothpaste Treatment in multiple settings if they feel particularly anxious or unsettled.

As a reminder, the goal behind this deep, slow touch is to help provide an orientation away from the outside environment towards the body, to better feel oneself and to feel the boundary of inside and outside. Through this practice we strengthen the first part of self-soothing, which is focusing and settling. When we are centered and relaxed, falling asleep is less of a challenge. The older children get and the more their awareness grows out into the world, the more they need to strengthen this quieting and centering capacity.

Some other ways to experience touch

Children may then continue their own touch experiences once they are tucked up in bed. They can initiate their own touch-boundary experience. For example, it can be helpful to move a child who has become independently mobile (crawling or walking) to a crib. Now there are four sides to lean on, push against, or snuggle towards. Those physical boundaries support touch-mediated self-orientation. Once a child has graduated from a crib, providing a bed that still has a headboard and a footboard, with one side of the bed next to a wall, offers continued chances to push, lean, or roll up against a strong boundary. For a kindergarten- or elementary-school-age child, a long, body-sized pillow can be helpful for snuggling. In fact, a child who piles all of their stuffed animals into bed so that there is almost no space for sleeping is probably seeking and needing touch throughout the night.

There are, of course, many forms of therapeutic touch. Occupational therapy for children often focuses on strengthening and regulating the sense of touch with techniques like large-joint compressions or dry skin brushing. With both of these, touch experiences are given which are stronger than normal, aimed at either the touch receptors in the surface of the skin (dry skin brushing) or the deeper pressure sensors in our joints (large-joint compressions). Weighted blankets and 'burrito' wraps around the limbs and trunk with a blanket (head and face kept free) can also be effective. For children with strong touch-seeking or touch-avoidant behaviors, these therapeutic supports can be very helpful for strengthening the experience of inner and outer world.

Whether introducing a calming experience of smell or a settling experience of touch, we can help children start to shift when they are stuck on the inward pathway. The introduction of a pleasing, gentle scent or slow, steady touch carries little risk. If it is not what the child needs, they will likely be indifferent towards it. On the other hand, when they are longing for support in their settling process, they will eagerly take it up. Once a consistent rhythm has been established, children look forward to these experiences. They offer helpful signposts on the path to sleep.

Quick reminders

★ As children grow older, the parenting task shifts. Our goal as a parent or nurturer develops into helping children feel their home (their body) and let go of the impressions of the day, through experiences of smell and/or touch.

★ Our job should focus on supporting the centering process, leaving space for the child to practice their own process of calming and feeling at home in their body. That second half is something they can only learn themselves.

★ A rhythmic bedtime routine, with a predictable progression for getting ready, signals that the day is coming to an end and that it is time for your child's nervous system to shift into a more relaxed and regenerative mode.

★ For touch-focused soothing, try the Toothpaste Treatment. Children who need even more experiences of deep, slow touch often benefit from a weighted blanket in their bed.

★ Seeking and receiving touch is a normal and healthy part of our human experience. See Chapter 9 for more ideas about the progression of touch experiences.

7. INDEPENDENCE AND BOUNDARIES FROM AGE 2½ ONWARD

The next step on the inner pathway provides yet greater capacities for centering and self-awareness. The sense of movement is one of the most inward sensing activities we need and use for calming.

Vision > Taste > Smell > Touch > Balance
> **Movement** >>> Well-being

Again, this is not one of the classically described five senses, but we depend upon it all the time. It helps us to know our movements in space, to feel the activity of our fingers, hands, toes, feet, limbs, and joints. It makes it possible for us to tie our shoes without looking directly at our laces the whole time, and to automatically turn out the light switch on the wall when we leave a room.

Part of the sense of movement is what's known as

proprioception: an awareness of the position of our body. Proprioception, at a basic level, is the difference between looking at what you are doing to guide an activity mainly through your vision (think of threading a needle), versus knowing where your limbs are from the *inside*, guided by the pressure and position receptors we have in our joints and muscles. To practice feeling this inward sensing, close your eyes and then touch your nose – this activity depends on proprioception. Such movement capacities are more than just geometric knowledge of limb position, however. They are part of a larger process of movement coordination, a task that depends on sensory receptors distributed throughout all the joints, tendons and muscles of our body, plus the activity of our cerebellum.

When children encounter new tasks, they often start by watching (vision), then move to encounter (touch), explore their relationship to new objects (balance), and then eventually become practiced enough to do the task more fluidly (movement). In time, with the practice of months, years, or even decades, we learn to vary the speed and strength of our movements.

In the same way that the sense of balance is more than physically feeling 'up' vs. 'down', or 'left' vs. 'right', the sense of movement is about more than just feeling the angle and position of our limbs. Both senses extend beyond their mechanical aspects: development of the sense of balance helps a child *feel their relationship* to their environment; development of the sense of movement allows a child to decide *how to interact* with their environment. For example,

if there is something I want to do, I might consider whether
I should do it now or wait until later. Is this a time to be
speaking or listening? Should I exert more or less strength?

Modulation of activity comes through this new sensory
capacity. It begins with adjustment of movement, but
eventually expands into all parts of life.

The sense of movement opens doorways for compensation
and adjustment. For a smaller child this might mean being
able to run across an uneven field without falling (adjusting
speed and balance while moving), or later being able to slowly
cut with a pair of scissors (squeezing the scissors to cut to a
certain point, but then stopping). For much older children,
movement allows them to play a musical instrument loudly,
then softly; or even to dance or move, in a coordinated
way, with a partner. The possibility for coordinated activity,
sensed and modulated *during* movement, comes about
through our sense of movement.

An additional element of movement in relation to the
other senses on this pathway deserves special consideration.
Here is Steiner's description of it:

> If we penetrate still further into ourselves we find
> a sense that inwardly reveals to us whether we are
> at rest or in movement. We don't only observe
> whether we are remaining still or moving simply
> by virtue of the external objects moving past us;
> through the extension or retraction of our muscles
> and through the configuration of our body insofar
> as the latter changes when we move about, we can

inwardly perceive to what extent we are in motion, and so forth. This happens through the sense of movement.[1]

A key phrase within this description from Steiner points to the possibility for a deeper kind of self-regulation, a capacity to 'inwardly reveal to us whether we are at rest or in movement'. How do we start to self-regulate?

First, we need to know both states, the opposite qualities of full movement and being at rest. Then, once we know these extremes, we can begin to explore the space in between them. Until we find that middle space we really can only choose between full activity or full rest. Toddlers predictably act this way: they are either fully engaged, into everything, continuously on the go, or else they are exhausted and soon fall sleep. They have not yet learned to self-regulate through the sense of movement.

How do children begin to develop that space in between?

Once again, the answer is through repetitive practice. For movement of the body, this means practicing being active and being at rest, muscle contraction and muscle relaxation. Every time we bend our arm, our biceps muscle must flex while our triceps simultaneously relaxes, and the opposite happens when we straighten our arm – triceps flex as biceps relax. Through repeated movements we learn to *know* both flexing and relaxing so that we can move between them. Gently pulling on an object (like a shoelace) requires both sets of muscles to be tightened, but not fully flexed. In a very practical sense, it is the difference between having only an on/off switch, which is more related to the sense of balance, or a dimmer switch that can be moved through a spectrum of intensity, made possible by the sense of movement.

Diverse expressions of movement emerge developmentally between 2½ and 4 years of age, the age when many children begin potty-training.

Learning to control bladder function follows the same pathway of sensory experiences that we have been exploring. It depends first on establishing a sense of boundary. Our experiences of boundaries begins with whole-body physical contact, such as being held or swaddled. As we develop more strength and mobility, we learn to initiate contact ourselves, mostly through our limbs, as a way of feeling ourselves, the sense of touch. Then comes a new step of awareness that differentiates our spheres of inner and outer activity, of sympathy and antipathy, the sense of balance. Awareness of our boundaries makes possible more specialized, physiologic awareness of where the bladder ends and the outside world begins. Eventually we learn to feel not just our boundaries but also the modulation of those boundaries: that is, when it's time to go to the bathroom and how to navigate that process in relation to other activities. This is the sense of movement.

This process takes practice. We start with on/off sensing, which is what happens when children realize they need to go to the bathroom and need to go NOW! but pee on the way there. The sensation of a full bladder comes and there is no possibility of holding it back.

A related, slightly older variation is when children realize they need to go to the bathroom, but tell you only after they have put on rain or snow pants, boots, coat, hat and gloves, or wait until you are in the car and have already pulled away from the house. With these second examples there is already more control, more modulation: the child can separate knowing about the need to pee from actually urinating, but the orchestration is not quite there. Planning ahead, going to the bathroom before putting on all the layers will likely still only happen with prompting from adults. In time, these capacities grow so that there can be true modulation of activity – from being able to *hold* urine until there is a bathroom available (a kind of rest), to *initiating* going to the bathroom now while there is a good opportunity (a kind of movement). Control of urine is one physiologic expression of children finding the space between activity and rest.

How long does it usually take to develop this sense of movement? Years. We continually refine our knowledge of this space 'in between'. It builds on the foundations of taste, smell, touch and balance. Some children move easily and quickly into this space of modulation with almost mercurial skill, while others struggle to really feel themselves deeply enough to be able to shift between movement and rest. Using the example of potty-training: many children learn how to be dry during the daytime between 2½ and 3½ years, but bed-wetting at night is not considered a medical concern before 5 years of age and is often still considered within the normal range of development up until the age of 7. To stay dry through the whole night, awareness of inside and outside must become so physiologically ingrained that a boundary awareness remains even when we are asleep.

Giving children freedom to explore

If we watch this progression closely, we discover a certain lawfulness in child development that helps us understand why a particular task or skill may be challenging for a child. **If a particular stage in a child's inner sensory development has not matured, such as touch or balance, then it will prove difficult for them to move on to the next stage, such as the sense of movement.** This pattern holds true for many different aspects of development. For example:

★ If a child has not received enough loving touch, exploratory touch, or self-engendered touch, being left free to take on more and more of the process as an independent activity, then they will not have developed a firm sense of being anchored in their own body.

★ If a child has not had enough opportunity to practice feeling the difference between left/right, up/down, forward/backward, with some accompanying risk of losing balance, then they will not yet have developed a firm sense of self and environment.

★ If a child has not sufficiently practiced moving between slower and faster, harder and softer, now and later movements, a skill we cannot directly teach them from the outside, then it will be difficult for them to navigate the dynamics of movement modulation or the shifting dynamics of social interaction.

This world, with so much time spent strapped into car seats, so many labor-saving devices and too many screens, blunts physical movement and risks stunting much more far-ranging sensory and social development.

> What can we do to aid this process? The best advice I know is to allow and encourage children to move freely and explore!

There is a very real, present-day danger that we are inadvertently robbing our children of the core building blocks for development. We don't do it out of ill will, but it does reflect a certain societal 'blind spot'. As a modern culture we over-emphasize the older, more intellectual expressions of the sensing activities that have been described. We may admire someone who has a secure sense of self, but rarely look to see how that person's senses of touch or balance actually give root to that stable sense of self. We tend to think that many self-regulating, emotional, and social capacities are techniques that can be easily taught or memorized, as if they are purely the outcome of a correct set of rules of behavior. But that's a fallacy.

It's a bit like believing that, because we have only ever bought oranges from a grocery store, whenever we want an orange then all we need to do is go out and buy one. That may be what most of us do, but it leaves out all the unseen elements that go into growing oranges and transporting them to the store.

Let's take this metaphor a little further. On our next shopping trip, we might find that there are no oranges, and we become so outraged by this that we demand to see the manager for an explanation. All this would show is how out of touch we have become with the seasonal cycles of growth and harvest times for orange trees. Maybe there are no oranges because they're not yet in season? Take the abstraction a step further and we could completely forget that oranges grow on a tree. Come to think of it, do you know what an artichoke, ginger root, or star fruit plant looks like? We tend to prize the end result, to want to enjoy the fruit and forget the process. Orange trees flourish because they have deep roots, soil, water, air, and sunlight. Nourishing those roots ensures continued harvest well into the future.

In the same way, healthy sensory explorations create and nourish the roots we need to really anchor and feel ourselves. We need those developmental roots to mature before we can properly sense the outside world or the other human beings. True social and moral health relates much more to these inward, foundational sensing capacities than to any kind of intellectual instruction or any set of rules.

As parents, teachers and caregivers, we need to become more like the farmers who care for the orange trees. We need an enhanced awareness of how important it is to nourish the roots of healthy sensory development. If we don't, we risk raising children who are all head, all intellect, without essential capacities for self-orientation, balanced judgment, and flexible action. Children need these skills more and more to adapt to the continuously changing conditions of this busy and unpredictable world.

Finding healthy boundaries for difficult behaviors

As children find increasingly independent means for self-orientation, self-soothing, and self-awareness, they also become more independent. This might seem like stating the obvious, but the process is multilayered. First, we see *movement independence* as a child learns to crawl, cruise, toddle, and eventually run away from you – 'I can choose where I want to go!' On top of that come layers of *emotional independence*, exercised by rejecting all manner of foods, requests, cautions, or corrections – 'I realize I am different from my environment!' These testing the limits of independence, as we've already seen (see Chapter 4 page 60), are not expressions of deeply held moral beliefs. They provide practice – 'What does it feel like to say "no"?' – and evolving social awareness – 'I can now let everyone know when I am scared or unhappy or disappointed.' This means that the inevitable episodes of exploration, chasing, insisting and ignoring are all healthy. They mark a child's dynamic shifting from one emotion or activity to another.

With the sense of movement and its possibilities for social modulation, a new kind of *social independence* begins. Movement allows children to go a step beyond refusal and ushers them into more nuanced processes of learning how to interact with others. For behind all the refusals, delays, and escapes, every child wants to find the best ways to be noticed and loved. Children just don't automatically know how to do it. It takes *social* practice.

Until there has been sufficient repetition and learning, a child's default behavioral patterns are usually either imitative – 'If everyone around me yells, then I will yell, too.' – or provocative – 'People notice me when I yell, so I am going to yell.' The latter aims to get a reaction and sometimes it works too well, with the parent chiming in and adding a little bit more yelling in order to stop the yelling. Sometimes it doesn't work as intended, with the parent choosing to pretend that there is no yelling happening at all and simply not responding.

The way a parent responds usually depends, to a certain degree, on the kind of interaction they themselves experienced as a child. We may model the exact same parenting pattern, imitatively or instinctively, that our parents showed to us, or we may intentionally try to do the exact opposite. Either way, it is good to be conscious of the pattern we are establishing.

Let's take the example of trying to parent a bedtime meltdown. Your child starts yelling and complaining when it is time to put on their pajamas or brush their teeth. Of course, no one really likes putting a whining child to bed. One parent may meet the meltdown by giving a strong boundary – 'Stop it, that's enough!' – in order to squash the complaining before it really ramps up. By contrast, a different parent may have decided long ago that confrontations only make the whole process longer and that it is easier to ignore the protests and move as quickly as possible through the process. In reality, we usually lean more towards one of these responses: either we confront, or we ignore.

Young children learn very quickly about these patterns and adjust their behavior accordingly. They learn to anticipate reactions, especially if they follow a predictable pattern. What happens if a child is always met with a strong boundary, especially an angry correction of behavior? The child learns that crying and complaining are not allowed. If a parent's response is sufficiently harsh, then the child's corresponding reaction may be to internalize the message that there is no place for complaints. Boundary interactions do have an important role. They are needed in unsafe or urgent situations when there really is no space for negotiation or protest. But if that's the default parental reaction it risks teaching a child that the best thing to do is to suppress or ignore feelings of unhappiness. In those situations, children will still feel anger, fatigue and sadness, but they will learn to not openly express those emotions.

> Inflexible boundaries send the signal that a child needs to stop and act differently, even if they are really tired, really sad, or really disappointed.

The opposite pattern can develop if a child repeatedly whines and complains, yet never actually comes up against a boundary. Protests, however loud or unpleasant, are always accepted or worked around. This pattern may arise out of simple parental fatigue, from being worn down and not wanting to fight the process anymore (a loss of patience and an angry boundary are also common with fatigue, too). But accepting a child's behavior can also be a consciously decided-on process. For some parents, avoiding a confrontation feels best because they have genuine sympathy for how their child is feeling. Parents understand and sympathize with their child's frustration. One result of this more sympathetic gesture is that because there is no confrontation, parents often end up doing most of the work. Putting on their children's pajamas or brushing their teeth for them is usually easier than arguing about it, even when the children could probably do it themselves.

Another possibility, if there is no consistent boundary, is that children learn to escalate. They get louder, provoke attention, refuse more, all with the goal of changing whatever it is that is making them unhappy. If there is enough protest, then bedtime takes so long that it becomes a de facto later bedtime, and the child can stay up for another 45 minutes. Leaving a fun party similarly becomes a long, drawn-out process because parents' repeated countdowns and warnings about getting ready to go, which are not then matched with a consequence, in the end just create extra playing time.

Both reactions – dominant boundary and accommodating sympathy – live mainly in the realm of the balance sense. Children like something or they don't like something. Parents react with a 'Yes' or with a 'No', with sympathy or with antipathy. Something is allowed or it isn't, much like the on/off switch of toddlerhood. So how do we move beyond these repetitive dynamics and begin to find the dimmer switch? As a child moves into the developmental phase of the sense of movement it becomes possible to build a middle space that allows for both expression of emotion and modulation of behavior. It has three steps: acknowledgment, boundary, and pathway (ABP).

The Acknowledgment-Boundary-Pathway Method

Acknowledgment

This means communicating to your child that you see them, using phrases like 'I hear you,' or 'Yes, I know that you are ready to go.' Acknowledgment builds a bridge for meaningful communication. You are saying to your child that you understand their struggle, see their enthusiasm, feel their emotion. 'I know that you're angry,' or 'I can see that you're tired (or bored, excited, restless, hungry, overwhelmed).'

Why is this step of acknowledgment important?

First, it signals that you are paying attention. Second, it helps break repeated patterns of escalation where a child has learned to get louder, wilder, weepier or more aggressive until someone reacts. Acknowledgment says, 'I am here, let me help you.'

> Where strong, rigid boundaries may teach a child not to express any emotions, lack of boundaries may lead to unfettered expression, escalation, even aggression. Once an emotional reaction begins, the horses start galloping and there is no one to hold the reins.

Boundary

This has a different role: it sets a limit. Expressing boundaries does not only mean you are being punitive; it is also an important way to share and define expectation. Voicing a

boundary gives parameters for how a child should interact
with others (including with you, as a parent). Sometimes the
boundary just needs to be stated by itself: 'You may not smash
things.'; 'You may not hit your sister.'; 'Screaming louder will
not get you what you want.'; or simply, 'Listen to me.' Clear
expression of boundaries can help frame an offer of assistance,
especially if it is paired with acknowledgment: 'I know you
are angry, but let's slow down and take some deep breaths,'
or, 'I know that you don't want to go, but we are not going
to fight about it.' Where acknowledgment is primarily an act
of feeling *with* someone, of sympathizing with them, voicing
a boundary creates form and separation, a gesture of stepping
away from a given behavior or interaction. Establishing
boundaries does not mean that one does not like a child. In
fact, communicating clear boundaries and expectations can
be a tremendous gift for a child who is socially disoriented
and looking for direction.

Pathway

Acknowledgment alone risks fostering patterns of escalation
because it doesn't require participation or cooperation from the
child. Boundary by itself risks building patterns of perceived
rejection and criticism, with a child learning it is better not to
express emotion or unhappiness. Together, acknowledgment
and boundary improve each other and create some balance.
But real kindness comes if we add a third step, the 'Pathway'.
This tells a child what they should do next in order to be seen,
heard, loved and met.

Acknowledgment and boundary frame the poles of behavior, much like the left/right, up/down, sympathy/ antipathy of the sense of balance. Pathway gives guidance for exploring the middle space of social interaction related to the sense of movement. Here are some examples:

★ For hungry nagging: 'We are all hungry (<u>A</u>cknowledgment) so let me finish setting the table (<u>B</u>oundary) and then we can eat (<u>P</u>athway).'

★ For bored nagging: 'I know that you are bored (A), but you may not look at my phone (B). We will be done in a few minutes (P).'

★ Aggression: 'You may not hit me! (B) I know you are mad (A), but we do not hit other people (B), and if you are that angry you can go outside and yell and stomp (P).'

There are of course many variations. Sometimes a situation calls for more acknowledgment, sometimes more emphasis on boundaries. The focus may need to be directed almost entirely towards differentiating between boundaries and pathway: 'You may not do this (B), but you may do that (P).' Use language that feels natural to you and appropriate to the situation and look to see if you are including all three elements. This method can help shift stuck patterns and provide a child with new orientation.

Bedtime meltdowns

Let's return to the example of a bedtime meltdown. The steps of acknowledgment, boundary and pathway outlined in the previous section can be particularly helpful for the process of getting your child into bed, especially if you find you are in a rut. On the one hand you want to help your child to feel safe and calm, yet you may also have reached, or long since passed, the time when it would be good for your child to take on more of the soothing process. We know that we want to acknowledge their discomfort, but also want to redefine the sleeping process, so that going to sleep does not need to be a long, drawn-out battle that exhausts everyone.

One secret is that **children are more flexible than we think they are.** If we set a clear intention, are consistent in the new rhythm or pattern, and include a pathway to show that we still love and support our children, good things can happen. As has been mentioned before, with a new routine it may well take a month for the change to become the new normal. In order to break a cycle, some parents will come up with a phrase that they know is fair and appropriate, have it ready at hand (even keep it on a piece of paper in your pocket for easy reference), and repeat it as necessary. Here is one for a bedtime that never ends:

> 'I love you very much (A), but it's getting dark outside, which means it's time for sleeping (B), and I will be very happy to see you and be together in the morning when the sun is shining (P).'

The phrase is clear and the part dealing with the boundary does not invite debate or discussion, it is the final statement for the evening.

It may not be heard so well the first time, especially when you are just introducing this kind of communication, so repeating it will likely be necessary. About the third or fourth time you need to say it, it can be even shorter:

'I love you (A), and I will see you in the morning when the sun is shining (P).'

At this point the boundary aspect comes not so much through words but by signaling that the time for talking is done – a verbal boundary. The emphasis moves more towards seeing each other in the morning – the pathway – with less and less acknowledgment.

After a while this kind of statement will most likely become boring for your child. That's intentional. Try not to explain or justify. It is a good, fair phrase. If you enter into discussion, then the boundary aspect of your communication falls away.

It generally shouldn't need to be said more than a few times, because then you, as the parent, need to slip away – a physical boundary. Will your child magically go to sleep if you do this? No, not necessarily. What you are doing is creating a new space, a middle space, for your child to practice self-regulation and self-soothing.

As adults we do this same kind of acknowledgment-boundary-pathway all the time, though probably more as part of our internal monologue and perhaps without such a formal structure. By the time we have made it to adulthood we have undoubtedly already lived through boring, challenging, uncomfortable or frightening experiences. In those situations we learned to practice modulation. We can say to ourselves: 'This is very uncomfortable/boring/challenging (Acknowledgment). I don't like it (Boundary), but this is only going to last for "x" amount of time, and then I can do "y" (Pathway).' Whether this relates to a boring meeting, a physical injury, an uncomfortable confrontation or a period of heightened insecurity, we exercise our own capacity for social and emotional movement. We sense ourselves and modulate our thoughts, emotions, and actions in real time. All of that is possible because of the sensory foundations laid at 2½–4 years of age.

That said, parenting and caring for young children is itself a major, repeated practice in both balance and movement. We start with certain patterns, certain inclinations of how we like to operate in the world – an experience of balance – and then meet situations that ask or demand that we shift and adapt – self-regulation, movement. It's a process that we never quite master. We never perfect it because we can't. By their very nature, modulation and self-regulation are perceptions of self that only unfold when we are in the process of moving and changing.

Sometimes, as parents, educators, or caregivers, we question our own knowledge and authority. We might feel that we don't really know enough to properly care for a child, so we spend a lot of time doing a tremendous amount of work trying to make them happy. We often find that our fuse is shorter than we would like it to be and lose patience with the whole process That's because we, too, must move between the polarities of acknowledgment and boundary and continually strive to find the right word, right activity, right understanding for each day.

We need to not only create a space for the children around us to practice physiologic and sensory movement, but also need to allow space for ourselves, as adults, to *practice* 'social movement' and 'moral movement'. It will not always be perfect, but we can learn from what does not go so well so that we can do it better next time.

And yet, we do have more than enough knowledge and experience to give good guidance. Think of a challenging social or emotional situation in your own life, perhaps with a loved one or coworker, and think how nice it would be if someone clearly communicated, first, that they hear you and understand what you are feeling (acknowledgment), then expressed what they cannot or will not do (boundary), and then shared what could be a path forward, together, towards compromise and collaboration (pathway). How amazing that would be! We can give the same loving offering, in appropriate doses, to our children as they are working to find their way in the world.

Quick reminders

★ Capacities for self-regulation grow out of the sense of movement. This sense takes years, even decades (or a lifetime?), to fully mature. It grows through practice.

★ Your child's sense of movement starts to awaken in important ways from 2½–4 years. This sense allows a child to both wait and hold back, and to initiate an activity before it becomes an urgent need.

★ Development of the sense of movement depends on the healthy maturation of the previous senses of taste, smell, touch and balance. It may be difficult for a child to work on their sense of movement if they are still continuously seeking taste or touch experiences as a primary means for orienting and soothing.

★ The Acknowledgment-Boundary-Pathway (ABP) approach helps frame space for your child to practice social and behavioral movement.

★ Young children, especially those 2½–4 years old, are too young to choose their own pathway. They cannot think through a situation without actually doing it. They benefit greatly when we can lovingly guide them with healthy pathways.

8. BUILDING WELL-BEING AND RESILIENCE FOR ALL AGES

Vision > Taste > Smell > Touch > Balance > Movement >>> **Well-being**

We now come to the inmost sensing activity along the inner sensory pathway. This is our sense of well-being. This is the sense that connects us to our own inner state of health. Most of the time our sense of well-being works so quietly that we do not even notice it. It's only when it falls out of balance, when we know that something isn't quite right with us, that we become aware of it. An inward signal tells us that we are about to get sick, or that we are too tired, too hungry, too over-stimulated. By contrast, the positive aspects of a healthy sense of well-being are contentment and an experience of comfort within ourselves.

Which organ relates to our sense of well-being? This is not so easy to pinpoint because it communicates such a broad sense of self. We can certainly say that a major component is the autonomic nervous system, which guides the functions and rhythms of our body that work right at the threshold of consciousness: heart rate, respiratory rate, pupillary dilation, sexual arousal, digestion, and urination. These are all realms where we have intermittent awareness, but which most of the time carry on without our conscious attention or direction. Our sense of well-being reaches beyond that threshold, too, connecting to the quiet, continuous functioning of many of our internal organs, such as liver, kidneys, endocrine glands and intestines.

It should not come as a complete surprise that the sense of well-being weaves through such a large domain, for as we have progressed along this inner pathway the sense organs themselves have become less spatially defined and more diffuse. The sense of vision is concentrated on our retinas, taste on the tongue, smell throughout the nose, touch across our whole outside boundary – our skin. Information about how our body is positioned in relation to the surrounding environment is concentrated in the vestibular canals of the inner ear, but balance, as we have discussed, is actually the larger sensing activity of the whole relationship between self and the outside world. The sense of movement similarly involves fine pressure and tension receptors throughout our joints and muscles, even as it extends beyond perception of joint position. It also makes possible motor coordination, social navigation and emotional modulation. Then we come to the sense of well-being – its quietness belies its essential role in self-perception. In truth, the sense of well-being connects us to the whole of our 'sleeping' inner world, to all the physiological, metabolic and homeostatic activities that keep us healthy and functioning on a daily basis.

Towards the conclusion of his description of the inward sensing pathway, Rudolf Steiner characterized the sense of well-being, or life sense as he called it, in this way:

> When do we enter the most into ourselves? When, within the general feeling of life, we perceive what we always have as our consciousness in the waking condition; when we perceive that we *are*; when we experience ourselves inwardly, when we sense that we are we. All this is mediated by the life sense.[1]

Our capacity to feel at home in ourselves, our fullest connection to the healthy life within us, arises through the sense of well-being. We sense that 'I am I'.

A primary task of childhood, especially during the first seven years of life, is connecting to this sense of well-being. To accomplish that we need the requisite time, space and sensory freedom to explore all the steps along the inner sensory pathway. Too often, we fail to see the importance of this process. Maybe we tend to overlook it because it's a quiet process and cannot be easily categorized or regimented. Maybe we fail to fully see it because the way it unfolds is always a little bit of an individual mystery. Whatever the reasons, we will raise happier, more resilient children when we properly nurture their sense of well-being.

In so many ways, our current society prioritizes capacities for sensing and taking in the world outside us over our more inward sensing capacities. We praise children for how well they see with their eyes, how carefully they listen, how much they remember. Those are measures of outer connection. But how well they then cope with the influences and demands of that outside world largely depends on the strength of their sense of well-being and how well they can correspondingly connect with, rebalance and re-orchestrate their inner world. There is a direct correlation between how well we orient and soothe ourselves along these seven inward steps and how well we can meet the outer world. When we are more 'comfortable in our own skin' – an expression closely connected to the sense of well-being – it frees us from becoming dependent on, and perpetually dominated by, outer conditions.

> Developing a healthy sense of well-being not only brings better rest and self-soothing, but also builds resilience.

Nourishing the sense of well-being

How do we nurture our sense of well-being? By supporting the quieter aspects of childhood: sufficient sleep, rhythmic eating, lots of free movement, and playful exploration, as well as protection from different forms of excessive outside stimulation that in today's world want to come too soon and routinely risk being far too much.

Getting enough sleep

We have already spoken a lot about sleep and soothing. Infants need plenty of external soothing, but over time children become able to take on more of the self-soothing and settling process. Hopefully, from reading the earlier chapters in this book, you will have gained a good idea of what that involves.

There are, however, two additional important aspects to consider in order to complete our understanding of sleep development: first, we need to be sure a child gets enough total hours of daytime and nighttime sleep, and second, that there is an early enough bedtime.

These are important because most adults do not, themselves, get enough sleep, and children need far more sleep than adults. Many behavioral and attention struggles are related to children not resting enough, and the problem is compounded when expectations for children's sleep are based on adult patterns. Here are common sleep recommendations for total hours of sleep (including naps):

★ **Newborns (0–3 months)**: 14–17 hours per day
★ **Infants (4–11 months)**: 12–15 hours per day
★ **Toddlers (1–2 years)**: 11–14 hours per day
★ **Preschoolers (3–5 years)**: 10–13 hours per day
★ **Elementary-school age (6–12 years)**: 9–12 hours
★ **Teens (13–18 years)**: 8–10 hours[2]

There are two observations to be made about these sleep recommendations.

First, because there is a range, we often interpret it to mean that if the length of time a child spends asleep falls within that range, then all is good. So, if an 8-month-old infant is getting 12 hours of sleep, including naps, and we see that the recommended range is 12–15 hours, then we feel everything is fine. But the reality is we don't know if a child is getting enough sleep unless we give them the opportunity to have 15 hours of sleep. It is better to aim for providing the upper end of the range and then see where your child falls. The lower end of the range is probably not going to be enough sleep for 90% of children in that stage of development.

How can you provide that much sleep time? Well, that leads to the second aspect, which is that most children do much better with an early bedtime. Toddlers do well with a 6:30–7:00 pm bedtime (some even like 6:00 pm). Many preschoolers thrive with a 7:00 pm bedtime. That means not starting to get ready for bed at 7:00 pm, but *actually getting into bed to fall asleep* at 7:00 pm. For a 4-year-old that likes 12 hours of sleep but does not regularly nap, a 7:00 pm–7:00 am sleep pattern is needed in order to get 12 hours of sleep. The main hindrances for providing this kind of rhythm are the work schedules of adults, as well as the temptations for after-school activities. But we don't build our sense of well-being through extracurricular enrichment. The deeper we go along the inner sensory pathway, the more a child needs 'down time' to practice that kind of sensing. The first seven years of life are the most important time for developing a healthy sense of well-being, which sets up life-long patterns for how we will sense and connect to the needs of our own body.

What if a child went all the way through childhood without ever really knowing what it feels like to be fully rested? What a loss. Learning to know when we are over-tired, and what it feels like to be well rested, are core aspects of the sense of well-being.

> We can't develop our sense of well-being through outer stimulation and instruction.

Eating regular meals

Just as we need time for both outward exploration and accompanying rest, all children similarly need rhythmic alternation between active eating and quiet digestion.

As part of the sense of balance, we discussed how consistent mealtimes help children to better anticipate and participate in their eating (see Chapter 5, page 66). Rhythmic eating actually reduces the need for parental reminding, herding, and cajoling of children to sit and eat. If breakfast comes predictably at 7:30 am each day, then at 7:20 am our body begins preparing for it with increased production of stomach acid and secretion of digestive enzymes. When children can lean in to a 7:30 am breakfast meal (or whatever time works for your family), they will be both more inwardly prepared to eat and more likely to want to sit down at the table.

Providing predictable mealtimes, as well as a dedicated eating space, like a dining room or kitchen table, helps frame the whole activity of eating. Whenever we can eat without distraction we meet our food in a much more complete way, better able to sense both the food and our own response to it. Small snacks throughout the day are admittedly quick and easy, but they keep a child bouncing between hungry and not hungry, with their blood sugar going up and down. None of those little snacking meals bring the full experience of feeling: 'I know my hunger, I see my food, my body is quiet enough that I am not distracted, and I can eat until I know I am full.' Learning to know when we are full – when we've had enough and feel satisfied – are core aspects of the sense of well-being.

Free movement and exploration

With each step along the inner sensory pathway, children increase the number of ways they can orient themselves in the world. More sensing doorways mean more potential paths to an experience of well-being.

It's helpful to remember that we essentially develop our sensing capacities through practice. During early body formation we grow the structures for vision, taste, smell, touch, balance, movement and well-being, but those are only the basic building blocks. We are born with two eyes, but research studies show that if one eye is mechanically blocked from receiving light the eye will become functionally blind; the brain does not connect to the eye and therefore cannot make use of any sensory input that later comes from it.

We therefore need to look and gaze day after day in order to develop a healthy sense of vision. We need to touch – thousands, millions of times – by grabbing, pushing, pulling, squeezing, sliding, and crashing. We spin, climb, lean, dip, walk a beam, hang upside down, and swing to develop a healthy sense of balance. We run, jump, catch, speed, slow, turn, stop, and start again in order to develop a healthy sense of movement. The nice part about free movement and exploration is that you don't need to set up a specific set of experiences. You don't need to hire a tutor, just give children the space and time to listen to the messages coming from their inner world.

Everyday obstacles to well-being

The next step towards better self-soothing will often unfold if we just get out of the way (see Chapter 3, page 46), and usually the answer for better calming is more free movement and exploration (see Chapter 7, page 98). What if the way to learn to be more inwardly secure is to be more outwardly adventurous? This requires the opposite approach from 'helicopter' parenting, which aims to make sure that everything is safe and secure before a child tries anything new.

Young children are highly imaginative; they love to play and explore, and we should let them. They are being guided by inherent wisdom. Hindrances arise when we – even out of the best intentions – limit their free movement or over-structure their activities.

Car seats and baby carriers

The world today is so full of labor-saving devices. We do not walk, lift, carry, dig or scrub the way we used to. We drive a lot. Children accompany us for much of that driving. That means that they sit in car seats, held securely in one position for their protection and security while we are driving. That protection is of course necessary, but it limits free movement. Even the various forms of baby carriers that can be strapped on to a parent's body – which are very helpful because the child can be with you while you have your hands free – also limit free movement. High chairs and other devices which hold a baby in a sitting or upright position over-emphasize one position, one activity. Ground or grass is much better. We artificially keep our children still in too many ways and this has a developmental consequence: it potentially blunts their capacity for self-soothing.

Over-scheduling structured activities

This one applies more to older children and takes a different angle on the developmental importance of free movement. It might even seem counter-intuitive when compared to the way in which a car seat obviously limits movement. The question is: what happens when children spend a lot of time in formalized dance classes or on organized sports teams? Hear me out – yes, there is movement, and yes, there is lots of practice moving the body. But there is a pervasive, societal confusion today that believes the earlier children begin to practice specialized kinds of movement, the healthier and more skilled they will become. The truth is that children need to first become comfortable with all kinds of movement and all manner of sensing activities.

The practice of specialized or formalized movement works best when it's built on a foundation of healthy, free movement. There needs to be lots of messy, imperfect, free, repetitive practice. You cannot do free movement wrong. We disrupt that when we place too much emphasis on perfecting very specific skills. The phenomenon of middle-school or high-school students burning out and quitting their very successful dance, lacrosse, or swimming activities after a decade of dedicated practice speaks to this risk. It is possible to become very good at an outer skill, yet still feel hollow on the inside.

Overuse of screens

If we were going to consciously create an activity that blunted overall motor development and self-soothing capacities by capturing attention and continuously looping it back to the sense of vision at the expense of the other senses, it is hard to think of anything more perfect than a smartphone. Whenever a toddler is kept occupied by looking at a game or movie on a phone or set in front of a television or computer screen, it creates short-term quiet at the cost of long-term capacities for self-soothing.

Screens are potent disruptors of both outer exploration and inner soothing.

The pervasive presence of screens in children's lives contributes, in a measurable way, to rising rates of anxiety in children. In fact, a very broad population study shows correlations between the number of hours of screen time and a proportionally increasing percentage of children who have 'been diagnosed with anxiety or depression'.[3] The same study shows that for groups of children aged 2–5, 6–10, 11–13 and 14–17 their scores on the 'easy child' index dropped (that is, children who were rated as being more difficult to parent) as their daily screen time increased, and that they were more likely to 'not stay calm when challenged'. The study includes one very special measure, which ties directly into our discussion of well-being. For children aged 2–5, it showed that the children who had more screen time were consistently less able to 'bounce back', 'often lost their temper', and were unable to 'calm down when excited or wound up'. Those are all measures of resiliency and self-orientation. They all relate to the presence, or absence, of a healthy sense of well-being.

If, as a child, your nervous system has developed in such a way that it is routinely dominated by a continuous flood of outer impressions from screens, how do you learn to feel comfortable and at ease with yourself? The answer is you may not.

So how much screen time should a child have?

I would very earnestly suggest that, until a child has really laid the foundations for a healthy sensing of taste, smell, touch, balance, and movement (which for most children takes until age 7), each hour of screen time should be balanced by 100 hours of free movement and exploration. That is a completely honest recommendation as a physician who deeply studies child development. Time on screens should be the rare exception, not the norm.

Limiting screen time is okay, precisely because outer world information and technology are moving so fast. Teaching a 4-year-old how to navigate an app will not help the child be a more successful adult worker in any meaningful way. The apps will all have changed. But young children spending hours a day on smartphones and iPads will be robbed of much-needed time to develop of a healthy sense of self.

The intense sensory diet of visual impressions seen on digital screens has observable, predictable, long-term effects. It stunts the sense of well-being and leads to children feeling increasingly unsettled when there is not a continuous supply of outer stimuli.

Unstructured time and play, with plenty of opportunities for freely walking, running, jumping, climbing, carrying and balancing, are all essential ingredients for the development of a healthy sense of well-being. The best gift we can give our children, right now, in the present time, is a greater sense of comfort, peace, and inner resilience.

Significant obstacles to well-being

Children come into this world with a strong, innate will to grow and explore. When it's time, they work to find the strength, coordination, and self-awareness needed for coming into an upright position.

Of course, it's important to remember that all development happens along a spectrum, so that the recognized milestone of being able to crawl at 9 months will be true for most children, but not all: some will crawl earlier, some later. As a general rule, however, if a child is not crawling by 12 months, then it is good to do a general survey of development to see if other areas are also proceeding slowly and consider whether additional evaluation or therapeutic support is needed. It's important to look to see if there are any physical, metabolic, cognitive, or sensory hindrances.

The basic process for assessment usually looks like this: **when a child shows challenges with venturing out to meet the world, you need to look more closely at the child, in concert with your child's doctor.** Said more simply: if outwardly directed exploration is proceeding slowly, look at a child's physical and neurologic health. Start at the center, with the child, and move outwards.

There may be rare children who are late to crawl because they have been held too much and haven't had enough floor time to gain needed strength and coordination. That's an unusual situation, because even if a child's physical environment is cramped or crowded, a child will work towards greater mobility and physical exploration. So for challenges with movement and mobility, the environment is not usually the source of the problem.

In contrast, **when children show challenges on the pathway of self-soothing, we need to look carefully at their environment.** If a young child's outer environment is hostile, unpredictable, frenetic or aggressive, the pathway towards a healthy sense of well-being can be strongly affected. In other words, if there are inwardly directed challenges with calming and orienting, don't forget to look outwards. Soothing capacities generally start at the periphery, and then move in. This direction and dynamic helps to clarify why some of the most dramatic disruptors of our sense of well-being come from our environment, as we will explore.

Very early soothing experiences of taste and smell depend on the presence of parents and caregivers. The actions of those adults are what bring calm. Infants are so open and connected to the world around them that they are hardly able to have a true sense of self. Infants' well-being is therefore strongly influenced by the activity, behavior, and presence of the those who care for them.

Addictive substances during pregnancy

We can see the influence of outside factors even before birth. During pregnancy, children in the womb are physiologically wide open to the world around them. Their 'world', their outside environment, is the mother's body and everything that the mother carries in her circulation. A child is continually being nourished (not through the mouth, but through the blood) through all that the mother brings into her system. This is generally a wonderful relationship, made possible by the great generosity of the mother's body, but it can leave the child vulnerable.

When there are intrauterine exposures to addictive substances, which by their very nature strongly manipulate our nervous system and shift the way that we sense ourselves, those substances can be tremendously disruptive to a child's just burgeoning sense of well-being. Drugs, as either stimulants or sedatives, bring one-sided sensations of self-awareness that are too intense and too early, and which may lead to long-term sensory and self-regulatory challenges. Children exposed to these kinds of substances in utero feel themselves too much, without being able to regulate the process. Before birth, children do not yet have access to the more normal postnatal soothing stimuli of taste, smell and touch. They lack those very pathways that make the transition into life more navigable and predictable. For children who experienced fetal exposure to drugs, working through the steps of inward sensing and self-soothing with dedicated care will provide essential footholds for growing and rehabilitating their connection to their own well-being.

Premature birth

A related vulnerability may come for children who are born prematurely. Here, once again, a child is exposed to strong outside influences, although now the environment comes through the portals of taste, smell, and touch. While this is still challenging, it is at least more navigable. Premature children are also pushed to feel themselves before their capacities for self-regulation and soothing are ready. The physical boundaries of inside and outside, such as the surface of the skin, are often still so delicate that they are challenged by anything but the gentlest touch. Bright lights, beeps and hums, IV lines, and unexpected handling all bring abrupt sensory awareness. Such unfiltered openness to the outside world creates a kind of sensory hyper-responsiveness. Children learn a form of protective vigilance. For this reason, prematurity presents an added challenge to a healthy sense of well-being for many children. From the moment they are born, neurologic patterns are built that prioritize sensations from the outside world (a self-protective reaction), even as the maturation of physiologic activities, such as respiration, digestion, circulation and blood sugar regulation, which usually occur in the late stages of pregnancy, are cut short. Children who are born prematurely often need extra time and extra protection from outside stimulation in order to build a full pathway to their sense of well-being.

Disruption in early life

Birth at term, after 37 weeks, allows time for more complete physical growth and physiologic development, but the sensory 'gates' of every newborn are still very open. Anyone who cares for a child in the first days and weeks of life will see the disruptive impact of noise, movement and commotion. To really nurture a newborn you have to go slow and be attentive. Parental neglect, due to illness, depression or abandonment, shakes the early foundations of the inner sensory pathway. An infant's well-being, at its deepest levels, depends on caregivers, and on being provided with the right experiences of taste, smell and touch to connect to their sense of well-being.

When there must be a change of parent or caregiver – even when it is done for the best of reasons, like adoption – that requires a reorientation on multiple levels. Anchoring experiences of familiar taste, smell, and touch must be found anew, even if adoption happens right at birth. It's important to openly acknowledge the dynamics of this reorientation, especially when tremendously loving care is being directed to the child from the outside and there's confusion about why a child may still be distressed.

That reorientation process takes time and invariably brings transitional experiences of confusion. It makes perfect sense that children who experience early life transitions or disruptions often take more time and require more repetition and more consistency to build an experience of safety. They need the opportunity to develop enough inner connection and activity to make up for the strong outer demands and impressions of early life.

Childhood trauma

Traumatic experiences, which can come at any time in the life of a young child, also bring imbalanced or premature sensing. These experiences are not easy or happy things to talk about, but they are a very real part of working with the inner sensory pathway to self-soothing. The long-term effects of Adverse Childhood Events (ACEs) have been well researched and described.[4] In the context of the inner sensory pathway, we can say that traumatic events, such as physical, verbal, sexual or emotional abuse, have recognizable effects on a child's sense of well-being. They are at least threefold:

★ **They disrupt a child's innate sense that the world is a good place and worth entering into.** All children have an inner call, an inner longing, to meet the world and to grow and explore, but abusive behaviors confuse that calling. Building self-orienting and self-soothing capacities require active exploration. Abusive behaviors threaten a child and usually blunt that exploration.

★ **With trauma there is little or no space to safely surrender to the outside world.** Children become hypervigilant, watching to make sure that they are not doing something wrong, or that an assault is coming. This pulls their attention outwards, again and again, to the surrounding environment. When a child has to devote tremendous energies to anticipating outside events, attention is continuously diverted from the inner pathway.

★ **Trauma can teach us that it is better if we avoid feeling ourselves too much.** When experiences of self are repeatedly combined with negative experiences and perceptions, such as pain, yelling, blaming, physical exploitation or sexual assault, then at some level it is often better to not really feel oneself. Connecting to an inner sense of wellness, experiencing ourselves inwardly through our sense of well-being where we sense that 'I am I', can be too much. Post-traumatic states frequently bring a kind of dissociative compensation, and we compensate for traumatic experiences by avoiding or not establishing a true connection to our inner world.

Rebuilding the inner sensory pathway

Speaking about those early life experiences – intrauterine drug exposure, extreme prematurity, early life disruptions and trauma – is sobering. The good news is that strengthening and supporting the inner sensory pathway aids recovery. Consciously supporting experiences along this pathway brings and helps to rebuild better resilience.

Granted, not all experiences affect individual children in the same way. Not all children born prematurely show long-term effects. Many children live beautiful, safe, flourishing lives with adoptive parents. People who experienced childhood abuse or neglect often go on to be tremendously loving and generous individuals. What then is the difference between feeling something as a shock versus a transition, experiencing something as traumatic versus unwelcomed? As a starting point we can work with this phrase: *trauma results when outside experiences create a lasting disruption along the inner sensory pathway towards well-being.*

When we can't find that pathway we must work to rebuild

it as best we can. We can start simply. Strengthening our own inner sensory pathway brings more resilience against the unpredictable assaults of the outside world. There is some paradox in the fact that the more we are overwhelmed by the outside world, the more we must call upon our own capacities for inward sensing and soothing.

What specifically nourishes our sense of well-being? Two good helpers are consistency of rhythm and trust in the world.

The importance of consistency and rhythm

The quiet, consistent, daily processes of hunger, thirst, digestion, fatigue, rest, and regeneration all come to consciousness through our sense of well-being. They provide connection to our inner world. They help us regulate and rebalance.

Like our other sense capacities, the sense of well-being develops through practice and repetition, though its orientation is somewhat different. It moves between our unconscious physiology and our wakeful consciousness. Its messages regularly spur us into action – for example, when it is time to eat, to drink and to rest – but then it turns back towards quiet watchfulness. It's a bit like a dolphin or a whale that briefly surfaces for a breath of air, but then swims, submerged, for much longer periods of time. It's a quiet, faithful observer. The activity of drinking a big glass of water (sensed primarily through taste and touch) might only take a few seconds, but our inward regulation of fluid balance cycles on continuously, day and night. Similarly, a quick meal might take less than ten minutes to eat (taste, smell, touch), but the ensuing digestive process to completely work through and transform that substance will last hours and days. We naturally focus on the conscious messages, believing that they are the most important part – but while a dolphin does need to come up for air, its main task is to swim.

Our sense of well-being connects to the depths of our unconscious physiology. It needs time to make uninterrupted 'dives'. We know this. A full night of undisturbed sleep will be more regenerative than an equivalent number of sleeping minutes divided up over many naps. Six snacks, even if they have the same combined calorie count, will not be as nourishing as sitting down for a full meal. For well-being to develop, it is the spaces in between the activities, and the meaningful work that happens beneath our wakeful consciousness, that deserve special attention.

Therefore, when we wake, drink, eat and sleep according to a consistent rhythm, we enhance the activity of all the inner processes connected to our sense of well-being. We digest better when a mealtime happens at the same time each day, rather than erratically snacking. We go to sleep more quickly and rest more deeply if we go to bed at a consistent time. Rhythm nurtures life.

These three foundational physiologic activities – eating/drinking, sleeping/waking, peeing/pooping – are not the right place for encouraging individual freedom of expression. These are the places for building a healthy foundation of self.

Supporting these rhythms is a core way in which we help children feel comfortable in their skin. And they are the main place we can start again when things become irregular, troubled, or unsettled.

One of the greatest supports we can give our children, to nourish and encourage the development of their well-being, is predictable eating, sleeping, and toilet habits.

Predictable life rhythms are, in fact, tremendously supportive for dealing with shock or trauma. Traumatic experiences specifically disrupt this inner sensing for what is needed, so we must work to retie the threads through rhythm and consistency. Sometimes we must start all over again and relearn when to eat, when to drink, when to rest, and when to get up. We recover more quickly if our sense of well-being has previously grown strong. Resilience in the face of adversity depends not just on the number of different pathways through which we can connect to our sense of well-being, but also on the richness and vitality of that sense. So, if you want to help your child build resilience, nourish their rhythms.

Trust in your child

We will finish our considerations for the sense of well-being with qualities of trust. Trust has actually come up multiple times, but in a quiet way. Did you catch them?

Parenting your child through these developmental stages is a dance. With each developmental shift there comes a certain moment when, after a lot of work to soothe, comfort, protect and guide a child, we have to step back and create a space for them (see Chapter 3, page 46). What makes stepping back so challenging is the fact that it may come just when we see our children 'wobble' – when they seem even less sure about orientation or safety. But if we trust in the developmental process and in our child's capacities for courage and growth, then rather than immediately jumping in and taking control of the situation, we will instead hold the space for our child to practice self-awareness. These trusting moments arise during 'restless' phases, when what had worked well in the past no longer provides the same comfort. The restlessness comes as a sign that a child (or even an adult – adults go through these cycles too) is ready for a new developmental step.

These moments are sometimes more of a test for us as parents and caregivers than for our children. We may not really trust the world. We may, in fact, have been working hard to protect our children from the insecurities and overwhelming feelings we experienced growing up. We may value the close connection we have with our children and be reluctant to give up that closeness so soon. Do they really need to become independent? Those are understandable feelings. There may not be a clear answer.

We can, however, gain orientation by asking: is a child doing something freely or have they become dependent on it? We all experience, right at the beginning of life, how a sweet taste like milk brings us calm. We can still enjoy that experience years later, appreciating a lovely dessert as part of a special celebration. Yet we recognize that something has become imbalanced if we always need to eat something sweet in order to find a sense of well-being. Similarly, being rocked or held as part of falling asleep is beautiful and comforting, but always needing a parent present in order to rest or sleep eventually becomes an uncomfortable crutch. Encouraging a child to move beyond a particular sensing activity for soothing really does not mean loss of that experience, just a broader repertoire of self-soothing capacities.

If we look once more at the stepping-stones of the inner sensory pathway for self-soothing, we can actually find a point of inflection, where an outer sensation becomes an inner experience: it is in the sense of touch.

Touch marks the transition point on this sensory spectrum where outer sensation becomes inner experience; where someone providing an experience of boundary from the outside becomes an inner process of orientation, of perceiving oneself:

Outer sensations

Vision > Taste > Smell > **Touch** >
                        Balance > Movement >>> Well-being

                                        Inner orientation

Outer guidance and reassurance, in time, become inner experience. If we don't allow for some 'wobble' and always try to correct and protect from the outside, it makes it more difficult for a child to progress much further along this pathway than the sense of touch.

Trust in life grows by learning about development. In fact, when you build a holistic view of development something quite unusual can happen – you become an enthusiastic developmental optimist! You risk becoming someone who goes around telling everyone they know about how the rhythmic unfolding of child growth and development shows there is great wisdom in the world, a great goodness. Very early in my medical career, one parent shared a story about the fatigue and worry of being a single parent caring for a 13-year-old child who had not yet slept alone through the night, not once. Bedtime had become long (2 hours), elaborate (many steps, lamps, sounds), and anxiety-provoking (for both parent and child). In desperation, the parent spoke with a kind, experienced doctor (not the author), who assured her that the child was ready to make a change and that it would be okay to let her struggle a bit and learn to sleep by herself. A few gentle natural medicines were also recommended, but the main ingredient was reassurance, which brought trust. After years of the mother fearing that leaving her child alone would bring trauma and fear, the 13-year-old learned to sleep alone, through the night, in two nights. Her mother stood up and told that story to the other parents who were gathered round so that they could be reassured.

Trust in the goodness and capacity of your child.

Quick Reminders

★ Your child needs a lot more sleep than you do as an adult and will likely thrive with an early bedtime! Remember that most of the children who are getting the lower end of the recommended number of hours of sleep are not getting enough sleep.

★ All children need downtime to build their sense of well-being. We can't teach it to them through outer stimulation or instruction.

★ Regular mealtimes will make it easier to get your child to sit down at the table and eat a full meal. It will help them digest better, too.

★ If children are allowed space and time for free movement and exploration, they will seek out the sensory experiences they need to develop their sense of well-being.

★ Strong, early disruptions can be very challenging to a child's sense of well-being. Children who have those kinds of experiences often need extra time and support to build their inner sensory pathway.

★ We can help children rebuild their inner sensory pathway if they have experienced trauma.

★ Goods ways to nurture and support well-being include consistent rhythms and trust in the world

Recommended steps

★ After reading this information, step back and look at the remarkable needs, challenges, and gifts of your child.

★ Create an affirmation for your child. What will help bring a healthy change? What do you want to do differently as a parent, and what will it bring to your child's experience of the world? What courage, or gifts, or peace?

★ Write down this affirmation for your child, as if you were writing them a letter. What do you hope to see bloom and blossom in your child?

9. STUCK SENSORY BEHAVIORS AND THERAPEUTIC APPLICATIONS

Exploring the steps and transitions that connect us to our sense of well-being doesn't just help with parenting, it also provides important insights and tools for therapeutic work. Many children who get lost or stuck on this inner sensory pathway exhibit strong sensory attachment, whether or not this is associated with deeper developmental or emotional challenges. Knowing the progression and timing of self-soothing provides a road map for helping a child take the next steps. We will now discuss two additional insights that help us to better parent, teach, or provide care for children who are stuck.

If a child seems stuck on a particular sensing activity, we can broaden and reorient their behaviors in two ways. Firstly, we can **encourage a more varied experience** of that same sensing capacity. For example, if a child is stuck on touch, we can give them the experience of many different kinds of touch. Secondly, we can **actively engage the next sense activity** along the inner pathway. So if touch is the problem, we can help our child engage with experiences of balance.

Let's take *thumb-sucking* as an example. It's a wonderful discovery when an infant finds a hand and starts sucking on a thumb or fingers. Now, suddenly, the child has a way to suck and soothe that does not depend on breast or bottle. If we look at thumb- or finger-sucking on the inner sensory pathway, it has definite elements of both taste and touch. It's a helpful and appropriate means of self-soothing for months or even years, but at a certain point it can feel more like a limitation than a boon – usually around the time a child begins to more actively explore the senses of balance, movement, and life.

How can we move our child away from a strict reliance on thumb-sucking? How do we diversify the possible pathways towards well-being? We begin by providing wide-ranging experiences of taste and touch. This can be as simple as providing crunchy or chewy textures on a more frequent basis – just make sure that the child has enough teeth to properly chew what you are giving them! Those textures help a preschool- or kindergarten-age child because they shift taste and touch away from stimulation of the roof of the mouth (which is what is mainly sensed during thumb-sucking) towards more mature experiences of teeth, tongue, and chewing muscles. We could also consider giving children thicker liquids to suck through a straw, like a milkshake or smoothie. This is an activity that requires stronger, more active sensations of taste and touch, and now includes lips and cheeks. We can also encourage more types of speech or song, as they give developmentally 'older' and more consciously guided ways to feel touch in the mouth. A kindergarten or elementary-school child who is still thumb-sucking may really like and benefit from tongue-twisters or whistling. These older-child activities – speech and whistling – bring experiences of touch, still located in the mouth, but now with less reliance on taste. That is the direction we want to go.

Another example of a kind of 'stuck' sensory seeking in younger children may be *genital self-stimulation (masturbation behaviors)*. There are some children who, as soon as it is time for nap or a rest, will immediately pop the thumb of one hand into their mouth and slide the other hand into their pants. Many concerns about masturbation are raised more out of social embarrassment than true concerns about a stuck sensory pattern, but some children are so dependent on genital self-stimulation that they rock, straddle, or rub their genitals to the point that it interferes with regular play and social interaction.

What can we do about this kind of repeated genital touching and stimulation? An important first step is to learn about normal types of genital touching and what are concerning patterns.[1] If we feel reassured that genital touching really centers around a dominant self-soothing pattern, we can follow very similar principles to what was described for thumb-sucking: that is, give more varied experiences of touch. We want to expand touch experiences beyond the groin area. If masturbation becomes a consistent part of a child's sleeping/soothing process, then giving broader deep touch (like the Toothpaste Treatment, see page 84) can be very helpful before laying down to rest. Encouraging more daytime touch experiences is also good. Activities like crawling, lifting, moving, and rolling all provide different ways for a child to feel their boundary. Usually, children are using genital stimulation as a way to ground and feel themselves. Genital self-exploration is quite normal in infants and toddlers. We just want to help children find diverse touch experiences so that they can develop flexible soothing patterns for different situations.

Beyond diversifying sensory experiences and encouraging developmentally more mature ways of working with a stuck sensory pattern, we can also support children by fostering experiences related to the next sense on the pathway. After taste comes smell, after smell comes touch, after touch comes balance, after balance comes movement.

Let's go back to masturbation behaviors, those that take place at nap time in a preschool or kindergarten classroom. In real-life situations, teachers have made consistent observations that children have been able to move away from genital self-stimulation for calming with more active balance practice, such as swinging or rocking, like on a balance board for example. A child may be stuck on one sensing activity because they do not yet know the next sense along the pathway. There is little risk involved in trying this out – healthy balancing activities are not going to hurt any child, yet they can provide significant support for expanding a child's self-soothing sensory repertoire beyond touch.

In the next part of this chapter, we will briefly revisit the steps of the inner sensory pathway with a view towards their therapeutic application. Some observations center around common behaviors, some around more extreme ones. They show the breadth of application for this expanded sensory view. Following the therapeutic advice for each sensory step comes a longer list of activities, chronologically ordered from the earliest patterns of young children to more advanced, self-directed activities of older children and adults. Hopefully these will give you ideas about the kinds of activities that will help a child make a developmental 'jump' to the next step on the inner sensory pathway and shift any stuck, unhelpful or damaging behaviors.

Taste

★ Taste calms and centers us, especially sweet taste. Always giving a child something to eat or drink when they are upset can build an over-reliance on taste as an anchoring activity. If what a child tastes is also predominantly sweet, that pattern often makes the over-reliance worse. Therefore, as a general dietary measure, make sure to *offer a broad range of age-appropriate tastes – sweet, sour, salty and bitter* (sometimes a bitter taste really helps anchor our taste, it 'sobers' it). Once children are ready for solid foods, they are also ready for a broad range of flavors. Just the encounter with different tastes helps broaden and diversify the ways taste can stimulate and orient us.

★ Diversifying the sense of taste can also be helpful when there is *a reliance on sweets* as part of disordered eating in teenagers and adults. The main point is not to reject or shame a longing – it is coming from a real place; it represents a real need – but help it be more flexible.

★ Some children with more significant developmental needs may *put everything in their mouth* far beyond the crawling and toddler stage: food, rocks, toys, chalk. This behavior can be about taste, but it may also represent a very young form of working with the sense of touch. Try encouraging somewhat older, more mature experiences for both the sense of taste and the sense of touch in these situations, like chewy or crispy foods, sucking on a straw, or blowing bubbles.

★ *Repetitive biting, whether a child bites themself or another child,* can be combined with other unusual taste-seeking patterns. In this case think about giving more mature taste and chewing/swallowing experiences. It's good to keep in mind that biting may not just be about outward aggression but can also be a way to feel oneself through taste or touch. The masseter muscles, which engage when we bite down, are the strongest muscles in the body – they can provide a lot of strong touch sensation!

Progression of sensing activities (many of these include an aspect of touch)

1. Taste of milk
2. Sucking
3. Swallowing
4. Taste of solid foods versus liquid foods

5. Experiencing different flavors: sweet, salty, bitter, sour, savory
6. Working with the texture of solid foods
7. Gumming
8. Chewing
9. Thumb-sucking
10. Sipping
11. Chewing hard or sticky textures
12. Speaking
13. Singing
14. Blowing (for example, blowing out a candle)
15. Blowing bubbles
16. Tongue-twisters
17. Whistling
18. Blowing (a musical instrument)

Smell

★ Some children show unusual behaviors when it comes to smell. *They seek out strong smells, whether from food, gasoline, cleaning products, or even the smell of their own sweat or stool.* This is a grounding behavior, probably a soothing behavior, albeit a very young one. We can offer children who are stuck in this way a diverse range of smells. We can make it a game, detective work to identify what something is, not just a behavior that will be chastised. This will help those children gain the additional experience they need for more fully developing the sense of smell.

Progression of sensing activities

1. Smell of a parent (milk, body odor)
2. Smell of place (bedroom, kitchen, grandmother's house)
3. Smell of familiar objects (blankets, pillows, stuffed animals)
4. Foods, with their aromas (smell is an important part of taste)
5. Soap, shampoos, detergents, body products
6. Aromatherapy, using an oil diffuser as a way to bring a particular smell into an environment
7. Therapeutic oils and creams (such as chamomile, lavender, or rose). Good-quality oils can be added to a bath as part of bedtime preparations, or a natural cream rubbed onto the body as a last part of getting into bed (rose and lavender can be very good rubbed over the heart).

Touch

★ Excessive or *destructive touch patterns* in children often represent a very strong need to stimulate their own physical sense of boundary.

★ Children who excessively *scratch their skin* when there are no obvious reasons to scratch, such as eczema or an insect bite, who *pick at scabs, chew their lips, pull out hair or bite their nails,* are often using touch as a compensation for emotional or social insecurity. We can therefore offer other, more positive, grounding, non-destructive experiences of touch, such as slow, deep pressure (through hugs or squeezes), crawling games, digging for hidden objects in a big bucket of dried beans, dry skin brushing, or working with clay.

★ *Skin-cutting and self-harming* in adolescents and teenagers can also be helped with this approach. Intense social insecurity, family disruptions, and bullying all threaten and undermine our sense of security. Proper medical support and counseling are essential in these situations to ensure safety, but positive experiences of touch, through massage with good-quality oils, loofah sponges, explorations with make-up or a new hair dye, or even something like the application of a henna tattoo, are all options for a healthy sensing and strengthening of the experience of boundary.

Progression of sensing activities

1. Birthing process (contractions and going through the birth canal)
2. Holding
3. Swaddling
4. Patting
5. Rubbing
6. Hugging, squeezing
7. Rolling
8. Crawling

9. Lifting
10. Carrying
11. Pushing and pulling (making contact)
12. Drawing with crayons (as a pushing and pulling activity)
13. Building
14. Tickling
15. Digging for hidden objects in a bucket of beans
16. Working with clay
17. Massage
18. Loofah sponges, dry skin brushing
19. Wrestling
20. Putting a body-sized pillow into the bed
21. Placing a bed against a wall and/or using a bed that has a headboard and footboard
22. Weighted blankets
23. 'Burrito' wraps, with a blanket wrapped tightly around the body (head and face kept free)
24. Hammocks (especially those with silk or vinyl that wrap around the body)
25. Artful application of a henna tattoo

Balance

★ Some children *cannot sit still*. They *continuously shift or shuffle* while standing, *lean and tip while sitting in their chair*, or *spin and twirl* while waiting in line. The best way to help them is to find engaging, age-appropriate ways to work with the sense of balance. These children are using balance as a way to anchor themselves in their body, and they are showing that they need a lot of balancing experience: walking a beam, swinging, jumping on a trampoline, walking on stilts, or learning to ride a unicycle.

Progression of sensing activities

1. Being rocked
2. Being picked up
3. Being carried
4. Rolling over
5. Sitting up straight
6. Pulling up to a stand
7. Walking
8. Running
9. Walking over an uneven surface
10. Climbing uphill, walking downhill
11. Spinning
12. Swinging
13. Balance beams
14. Rocker boards
15. Somersaults
16. Teeter-totters or see-saws

17. Merry-go-rounds
18. Balance bikes
19. Playing hopscotch
20. Trampolines
21. Stilts
22. Bicycle riding
23. Skateboarding
24. Unicycle riding

Movement

★ Some children's **inability to be still or to come to rest** stems from their need to regularly be in motion. They best connect to, and sense themselves, when they are actively moving. Allowing for more movement is a natural support, but not all movement is equal. Movement that comes as part of a practical task works better because it allows a child to bring consciousness into the movement over and over rather than letting the 'galloping horses' of unguided movement run free. For an older child, movement activities that are done with partners work well. If you really want to challenge someone who needs to be in constant motion, help them learn to juggle (movement to the extreme!). Then juggle on a unicycle (now with a whole lot of balance).

Progression of sensing activities

1. Walking
2. Running
3. Jumping
4. Climbing
5. Eating with a spoon or fork
6. Pushing (against resistance, like opening a heavy door)
7. Pulling (against resistance, like holding open a heavy door)
8. Catching
9. Pedaling (a tricycle or bicycle)
10. Slowing down when we go too fast
11. Speeding up when we lose momentum
12. Sawing
13. Shoveling
14. Tying a shoelace
15. Zipping
16. Buttoning
17. Weaving
18. Juggling
19. Actively listening when we really want to speak
20. Changing a habit

Well-being

We connect to our sense of well-being every time we center ourselves, every time we listen to our own needs, every time we feel that we are ourselves ('I am I'), as a counterbalance to the demands and impressions of the outside world. Common examples include:

1. Relax into sleep
2. Relax after a busy activity
3. Calm after a disappointment
4. Calm when we feel disoriented
5. Calm after a shock or surprise
6. Know when it is time to sleep
7. Know when it is time to eat
8. Know when it is time to go to the bathroom
9. Stay seated to eat a full meal
10. Sense when we are full
11. Sense when we are over-extending ourselves
12. Sense when we are overwhelmed
13. Consciously do some breathing techniques to promote relaxation
14. Do a 'body scan' for relaxation
15. Meditate
16. Focus on the present moment
17. Cultivate gratitude

10. COMMON TIMES OF ANXIETY AND TRANSITION

We've talked in multiple ways about the soothing patterns of newborns, toddlers, preschool- and kindergarten-age children. Childhood is full of self-soothing adjustments and disruptions. An additional key aspect is that we don't just take continuous steps forward. We often hesitate, or even take a step or two backwards, as we adjust to a new situation. It's helpful to recognize that during these moments of transition, as we change our sensing/soothing patterns, there are often observable behavioral stutter-steps.

> Developmental stutter-steps happen quite predictably at the threshold of any change. We come into an expanded awareness of something new. The world gets a little bigger. It's exciting, but we waver, thinking 'Is this really the right thing to do?'

Consider the exciting exploration that comes with learning to crawl. Usually 9- or 10-month old children will crawl away with enthusiasm, but at a certain point they stop, look around and realize, 'Oops! That's a little too far away from my parents for comfort.' Then they come back for reassurance. A few minutes later they are exploring again, maybe a little further this time, but still not too far. 9–10 months is also the stage, not coincidentally, that children typically develop a fear of strangers. That's a stutter-step: they feel a new independence and curiosity, combined with a new awareness of aloneness. Newly crawling children are a lot like ships that leave their harbor to explore in gradually larger loops, but still need lots of reassuring voyages back home to check in.

Let's now think of an older child, one who's excited at the chance to sleep away from home for the very first time. How adventurous and simultaneously frightening that experience can be! The overnight feels wonderful until sometime around bedtime when the child gets suddenly terribly homesick, so lonely, with flooding tears. A parent may even have to come and bring the child home. We are excited, we adventure, and we are exposed.

Even as adults we experience stutter-steps, with house moves, new jobs, losses and changing relationships – moving forward, backward, forward, backward, until through enough repetition we grow comfortable with the new situation. It takes practice before it begins to feel navigable. In the interim, when we are still not sure about the newness of our experience, we naturally incline back to what was previously known. We gravitate to the things that helped us feel safe and secure in the past.

When we carefully observe these patterns, we see that there are really a whole set of developmental milestones, not only for movement, speech and socialization (the mostly commonly described), but also for changing sleep patterns and for self-soothing. The following pages show a table that combines those well-established milestones for gross-motor skills, fine-motor skills, language and social interaction with common changes to sleep patterns. Then on the right-hand side are added observable milestones for soothing and self-orienting. This new category for self-soothing 'milestones' – based on the inner sensory pathway – is less fixed. There is naturally greater variability and individual timing for these changes, yet they do follow a characteristic unfolding over the first years of life. Combining all of this together, we can see how exploratory outward steps parallel and are matched by new inward steps of perception and anchoring.

As we step further out, we must also necessarily step in. That mutual sensory exploration builds resilience.

Developmental milestones, sleep patterns and self-soothing in the first 5 years[1,2]

Age	Gross Motor	Fine Motor	Language
1 month	Lifts head momentarily.	Fixates on human face and follows with eyes.	Responds to sound by blinking, crying, showing a startled response.
2 months	Raises head and chest when lying on stomach.	Makes smoother movements with arms and legs.	Coos and reciprocally vocalizes.
4 months	Rolls from tummy onto back.	Opens hand, holds own hand, grasps rattle.	Smiles, laughs and squeals.
6 months	Begins to sit without support.	Transfers objects hand to hand; brings objects to mouth.	Babbles reciprocally, responds to own name.
9 months	Creeps, crawls, moves forward by scooting on their bottom.	Uses pincer grasp; finger-feeds.	Imitates speech sounds (nonspecific 'Mama/ Dada').
12 months	Pulls to a stand; cruises.	Can voluntarily release items; feeds self with fingers.	Speech sounds: 'Mama/Dada', plus 1–3 other words.

Social	Sleep	Self-soothing
Responds to parent's face and voice (by 1 month).	Sleeps most of the time; awake for a maximum of 1–2 hours.	When crying, can be consoled by nursing (**taste**) or being held (**smell**, **touch**).
Begins to smile; tries to look at parent.	Timing of naps still unpredictable.	Can briefly calm themselves; may bring hands to mouth and suck on hand (**touch**).
Recognizes parent's voice and touch.	Sleep cycles become longer.	Practice of self-soothing begins for sleep to last for more than the usual 50-minute sleep cycle.
Identifies object or person as unfamiliar.	Naps often consolidated into three periods.	Starting solids, so the sense of **taste** begins to shift (no longer so closely connected to sleep).
May be afraid of strangers, responds to own name.	Begins to notice when parents are not there, may wake to check.	Crawling brings stronger experiences of **touch**. Children become more independent in terms of their **movement**.
Has favorite things or people; cries when parent leaves.	Many children go to two nap periods; routines become more important.	Standing allows them to independently **balance**.

Age	Gross Motor	Fine Motor	Language
15 months	Walks well Independently.	Stacks two blocks; begins to use a cup.	Vocabulary of 3–10 words.
18 months	Walks quickly or runs stiffly.	Uses spoon; spontaneous scribbling.	Vocabulary of 15–20 words; makes sounds with changes in tone (more like speech).
2 years	Kicks ball; can go up and down stairs one step at a time.	Uses fork and spoon; points to some body parts.	Has a vocabulary of at least 20 words.
3 years	Pedals tricycle.	Copies a circle.	Carries on conversation using 2–3 sentences.
4 years	Hops and jumps on one foot.	Catches a bounced ball most of the time.	Tells stories.
5 years	Skips with alternating feet; swings and climbs.	Draws a person with 6 body parts; can count on fingers.	Tells a story using full sentences.

Social	Sleep	Self-soothing
Understands simple commands.	May no longer need a morning nap; good to try an earlier bedtime.	Free exploration continues. Many children are ready to shift from **taste** as a pathway for soothing to go to sleep to **taste** as part of exploration (putting everything in their mouth). Important practice of **smell**, **touch** and **balance**.
Explores alone but with parent close by; shows affection, kisses.	A nap is still needed, waking in the night may start again.	
Plays mainly beside other children, imitates adults.	Bedtime battles begin. Now is often a good time to move from a crib or a cot to a bed.	Children become aware of the difference between inside and outside (between self and the world). Potty-training can begin. **Balance** finds both physiologic and social expression.
Shows a wide range of emotions, understands the idea of 'mine' and 'his' or 'hers'.		
Enjoys doing new things; imaginative play.	Some children may stop napping, but still need a consistent time to rest in the afternoon.	Parenting task is more to set healthy rhythms and patterns, rather than to make a child fall asleep. **Balance, movement, well-being**.
More likely to agree with rules; wants to be like friends.	Most children stop napping.	Enjoys feeling capable; eager to explore new activities and capacities. Enhanced experience of **movement** and **well-being**.

Considered as a whole, we can see that these changes are not just about strength, coordination and sensing, but really about an evolving sense of self. We become broader and deeper in terms of capacity and confidence. We can describe it in this way: we are born with certain physical organs, such as bones, muscles, ears, eyes, nerves and so on, then, as a secondary step, we learn to make use of them. It's not an automatic thing that we know how to use what we are given – quite the opposite; it takes years. But once we have a working understanding of our bones, muscles, ears and eyes, we take a third step, and that is we work to individualize them. We make them our own. We could think about this progression in terms of having legs (birth), learning to walk (12–15 months), and then having a distinctive, individual gait (elementary school to teens). Or, being born with lips, tongue, teeth and cheeks (birth), learning to talk (12–36+ months), then having our own distinctive voice and special way of speaking (elementary school to teens to adulthood).

It takes time to grow a whole human being; we are not like an automobile that is ready to run once you put all the pieces together. An essential misperception stems from the idea that once we have all the parts, we should simply do things as early as possible, a view that leads us to the opinion that children are basically just miniature adults. They aren't.

Awareness needs to come in predictable waves, at predictable times, so that we can, in fact, weave back and forth between outward changes and greater inner connection and self-perception.

★

Knowing about the timing of developmental shifts that continue beyond the first five years of life can be extremely helpful, particularly because they are now so routinely misinterpreted. Children are too often being diagnosed with an anxiety disorder or depression, probably because we don't know how to deal with the way they are expressing the changes they are undergoing. This does not mean that we should leave children alone to suffer, rather that, as a society, we need to learn more about how to proactively work with processes of change. We tend to think of growth as always being about adding new skills, new knowledge, new possessions or new accomplishments. But *dissolution* and *reorientation* are also key ingredients. To grow forward into the future, we must let go of some of the patterns of the past and this does not happen with the flip of a switch. There needs to be a period of transition, and these periods are exactly where we would expect to see a stutter-step, when a child (still mostly unconsciously) recognizes that old patterns are no longer sufficient, but they do not yet have enough experience with new capacities to feel comfortable.

We should understand these predictable biographical rhythms as essential times for transformation of self-experience and not fear them too much. These thresholds have been deeply studied and well characterized within the streams of Waldorf education, Camphill programs for curative education and social therapy, and Anthroposophic Medicine, though aspects of them surely also live in other holistic streams of education and healing.[3]

One striking insight provided by this approach is a certain pairing of developmental windows. New steps of independence appear first more inwardly, on the level of how we experience ourselves, then later more outwardly, in terms of how we experience the environment. Some of these thresholds will be familiar, whereas others will perhaps be quite new. But once you notice them it can become hard to unsee them, as they play such an important role in the life of children.

Transitions of independent growth and thought

We have already looked in depth at two of these developmental windows: birth, when taste, smell and touch make a big entrance, as well as 2–3 years of age, where bigger steps of self-regulation enter in through growing capacities of balance and movement. We will briefly look at birth once more, though now as a physiologic stutter-step that leads towards a more independent physiology.

Birth

As we have discussed, with physical birth the warmth, nutrition and protection a child has been bathed in for nine months falls away. Suddenly each child has to breathe on their own, learn to nurse, open their eyes and see, hear, touch, pee, poop, and maintain their own warmth. Birth is a huge developmental and physiologic shift! We don't usually think of newborns as having an anxiety disorder because we recognize right away that they are tremendously sensitive beings and need lots of protection. Our care instinctively goes towards soothing them and helping them adjust to new rhythms of eating, sleeping, and breathing.

Growth activities really become the child's own. These activities continue to mature so that by 7 years of age, many of the body's largely unconscious regulatory processes (digestion, movement, sleep) have become well-practiced. In many ways, the first seven years of life is the most essential time for developing and strengthening the inner sensory pathway towards a healthy sense of well-being, a process that begins with birth.

What happens?

★ Birth marks a major step in physiologic growth and independence. This is a major transition – a stutter-step for being in the world in so many new ways.

★ Once a child is delivered, activities of growth and nutrition no longer depend on the mother's body. A child can be cared for by birth parents, adoptive parents, or other caregivers (which was previously not possible).

★ The process of exploring the inner sensory pathway towards well-being begins.

What to do?

★ Newborns need great protection. In truth, it feels appropriate to consider children in the first weeks and even months of life as experiencing separation anxiety after having left all the warmth, nutrition and protection they experienced during pregnancy.

★ An infant's senses are wide open to the world, without the possibility of ignoring or prioritizing what they take in through sense impressions. They are easily vulnerable to sensory overwhelm.

★ Supporting rhythms of eating, soothing and sleeping are the main parenting task, as inward capacities for self-soothing exist only in seed form.

★ Caregivers must gently and consistently provide needed experiences of taste, smell, and touch from the outside for the child to develop experiences of well-being.

6-7 years

This age rounds off consideration of the major physiologic shift that occurs with birth and marks a further maturation. 6–7 years is marked by a distinctive growth step: the appearance of adult teeth. Losing baby teeth can start earlier (sometimes around 5 years of age, or even younger), but just losing teeth without having adult teeth ready to grow in does not really signify this developmental step. We know that something has fundamentally shifted when new teeth appear from the inside. This is also the age when the '6-year-old' molars grow in, another mark of this developmental threshold.

The eruption of adult teeth shows that a certain level of physiologic ripeness and maturity has been achieved. By this time children can generally eat, sleep, move, dress, bathe, run, and listen with confidence. They are ready to move out into the world in a new manner, ready to take in and 'digest' the world in new ways. They become more interested in peers and friendships. They are no longer so imitative, a sign that they are less needful of and less dependent on their parents and caregivers. Many parents themselves experience a shift, a release at this stage, as the intense parenting energies needed to nurture a child lessen.

Children show that a change is happening not just on a bodily level but also on a cognitive level. They show this by demonstrating new ways of thinking: they begin to think abstractly. Children who have been allowed to go through the first years of life without excessive stimulation or abstract instruction exhibit a wonderful curiosity at this age. You can see that they are really growing new thoughts: 'What does that mean? What does that sign say?' Children start making new associations so that letters and numbers and all manner of symbols have newer, deeper meaning. Thinking is no longer so literal, so connected to the physical body. Thinking becomes 'body-free' in that a child can now work things through in more flexible ways, such as doing addition problems by mental math instead of always needing to count it out on the fingers. Children also become better able to plan and think something through instead of always having to physically act it out.

Meaning becomes more flexible. Children at this age

also love to explore their new thought capacities through puns and jokes. Up until this time a child might imitate the pattern of a joke, such as knowing the sequence for a knock-knock joke, and at the end just inserting a random word and laughing – because that is what they have seen. Previously they were mainly imitative without really understanding how a joke works. They just enjoyed knowing that the knock-knock joke pattern signified a time to laugh and so they repeated that pattern. But now they can actually begin to hear the differences in meaning, moving words and sounds around in their mind in order to make new connections. They can hear the difference between 'Aren't you glad?' and 'Orange you glad?', or a pun like 'Lettuce be friends,' and want to tell lots of people about their new discoveries.

On many levels, 6–7 years of age is a time to celebrate new growth and new ways of understanding the world. It is, however, a common time for children to regress or stutter-step. Some children will wet the bed after being dry for a number of years. Some will get stomachaches that come in anticipation of going to school but are absent on weekends. Some may want to again crawl into their parents' bed in the middle of the night.

This is a good time to give gentle reassurance and celebrate new explorations. If things are too much, go slow and make sure your child is getting enough rest. Remember that elementary school children still need 9–12 hours of rest, so if things seem rough, try to provide a full 12 hours of sleep.

What happens?

★ This is a major transition in terms of growth of independent *thought*, a stutter-step for cognitively understanding the outside world in new ways.

★ Physiologically, children begin to lose their baby teeth and adult teeth grow in, '6-year-old' molars emerge, limbs lengthen and body proportions shift.

★ At this age children start to think abstractly. Their observations of the world change; they are curious about what things mean.

★ They do not imitate adults as instinctively as they used to.

★ Thinking is no longer so connected to their body; they are no longer such concrete or literal thinkers.

What to do?

★ It's important that there are rhythmic alternations between independent activity, like the school day, and quiet, predictable time at home.

★ Considering the world in new ways takes a lot of energy. If you see regressive behaviors, set an earlier bedtime.

★ Many sensitive children are working incredibly hard to do everything properly and not be caught off guard during the school day, and they come home completely worn out. After-school or evening meltdowns are a sign of being overwhelmed or over-tired, even when these new opportunities to explore and learn are exciting.

★ Celebrate new capacities, new strengths and awareness. Children at this age often like to hear stories about what they did when they were babies – a way to revisit an earlier way of being that they can feel is changing.

★ Your parenting job at this point is to give direction and rhythms, guidance and reassurance.

★ Suggested bedtime soothing process: 35% parent (you are setting the stage for sleep), 65% child (but it is no longer your job to make a child fall asleep).

Transitions of emotional and social connection

The developmental shifts that occur at birth and at 6–7 years of age center around evolving processes of independent growth and independent thought. The developmental thresholds that come at 2–3 years and 12–14 years are more about sensing and emotion.

2-3 years

We've already looked at this developmental window in relation to the sense of balance (see Chapter 4, page 58). The physiologic capacities for feeling left/right, up/down, forward/backward become more practiced. Potty-training also often becomes possible in this window, as a child begins to feel the difference between inside and outside.

The larger social and emotional changes seen at this age grow out of a child's realization that they are distinct from their surroundings. They experience the first glimmers of a new boundary between 'what is me' and 'what is not me'. This is classically a time of children practicing saying 'No' to all kinds of things, not so much because they hold deep moral objections but because they are practicing saying 'No', practicing being distinct. They need to feel what it is like to be separate. They need to alternately practice sympathy (in the sense of coming together with something) and antipathy (as separating away from something). They do this swinging back and forth because the border between inside and outside is still being created and is not yet firm. We can observe how this border shifts, because the thing that a child emphatically said 'No' to five minutes ago may now be just fine. Refusals are a practice in process, not principle.

What happens?

★ A major transition time in terms of independent *emotional* and *social connection*, a stutter-step for starting to feel how one can be separate from the environment.

★ Children at this age are building the foundations for a healthy perception of their emotional and social self, which will find its next evolution at puberty.

★ This is the age of the Terrible Twos (with first glimmers appearing as early as 18 months).

★ Children at this age like to practice saying 'No!' It is not an expression of logic or morality. They are practicing feeling their own boundary.

★ They also start to potty-train, which helps them to feel the border between inside and outside.

★ This is an age when children can become quite stuck on a younger soothing pattern, particularly taste or touch. That regression points to the fact that they are looking for new ways to orient themselves in the world.

What to do?

★ Allow for explorations of boundary. Don't take it personally when a child rejects what you so lovingly offer. It doesn't mean they don't love you! Focus on being consistent.

★ Encourage participation with daily rhythms and activities: toileting, eating, getting dressed, expressing needs, communicating together.

★ Provide rhythmic 'signposts' to help signal when something is going to change, such as: consistently sitting at the table at mealtimes (now it is time to eat); speaking a verse or poem at bedtime, or always singing the same short song (now it is time to sleep).

★ Rhythmic activities help a child know what comes next and how to participate. They offer the pathway for a child to become more involved in the world.

12–14 years

The further evolution of emotions and social connection comes with early adolescence, which marks the end of a second seven-year cycle.

There are, of course, lots of outer changes – notably all those physical shifts associated with puberty. The forces of differentiated emotion experienced at 2–3 years of age (sympathy/antipathy, yes/no, happy/sad) now find expression through the differentiated physical development of secondary sex characteristics, such as breast development and widening of the hips and pelvis in girls, and change of voice, growth of facial hair and widening of the shoulders in boys.[4] These changes mark the body's shift towards more 'polar' qualities of female and male reproductive physiology. Most adults remember the challenges of this stutter-step towards adulthood, with a changing body that may or may not feel comfortable. The timing of these physical changes varies, with it now becoming increasingly common for girls to experience pubertal changes well before 12 or 13 years of age. The broader maturation of social and emotional forces, however, still typically find expression around the end of the second seven-year period.

The end of the first seven-year span brought readiness for more independent thought activity (marked by adult teeth). The end of the second seven-year cycle, during puberty, brings continued physiologic independence, plus a powerful social reorientation. Young adolescents want to do their own thing, find their own interests, and spend more time with peers. Reproductive maturity naturally means that primary social and emotional dynamics move away from the parent–child relationship towards others.

Swinging emotions are everywhere. It can feel as if new forces of social orientation, both good and bad, well up into consciousness overnight. A young adolescent frequently feels so deeply connected to a friend (or a crush, song, or inspiration) that it takes hold of nearly all waking consciousness. But then, just as abruptly, adoration or obsession may end, bringing such utter isolation or loss that it is hard to even know how to be in the world. Obsession with a craze or crush (sympathy), alternates with loss or feelings of rejection (antipathy).

This new wakefulness of feelings brings gifts. As forces of rejection and rebellion need to emerge, helping a young person find healthy outlets for this 'birth' of independent feeling makes the transition easier. This is such an important time for finding new role models and identifying new aspirations. Artistic sensitivity awakens for personal style, music, movies, and all kinds of popular culture. Encouraging different forms of expression helps ground and orient the sudden swinging of feelings, such as new ways of dressing or finding a new skill or hobby.

As they approach 14 years, some children will speak with great fondness and a kind of nostalgia for what their life was like as a younger child. The outside world, with so many social pressures and dynamics of identity, attraction, and isolation, often feels overwhelming. Disorientation is normal as the more sheltered consciousness of childhood is left behind in order for a more independent sense of self and social connection to come forward. Things get off balance precisely because adolescence is the time when emotions stop being so imitative. They are freed so that they can become one's own. It's a needed evolution, as the more physiologic boundary building of 2–3 years plays out on a much larger social and emotional level.

What happens?

★ A major transition time in terms of *emotions* and *social connection* with the outside world, a stutter-step for feeling how one should independently relate to the outside world.

★ The body begins to change with the arrival of puberty: growth spurts, voice changes, breasts, periods, and body hair.

★ Social awareness expands: awareness of self and peers, awareness of connection to other people and isolation (separation) from them.

★ The physiologic rhythms of 12–14-year-olds become more independent; the inherent rhythms that helped them know when to eat, when to sleep, and when to get up are cast off.

★ A kind of teenage physiologic imbalance emerges as the model of parents and other adults is rejected in favor of a more independent exploration.

★ Artistic awareness and expression take on much greater meaning through music, clothes, hair, make-up, style, fads, and general non-conformity.

★ Frequent swings in terms of emotion and social connection.

★ A need to actively seek new things, while simultaneously rejecting lots of other things and wanting to be different from others.

★ What might have seemed so settled in older childhood (at 10 or 11 years) now becomes chaotic, all so that an adolescent's sensing and emotional capacities can truly become their own.

What to do?

★ Boundaries are pushed (although they are still very much needed). Rebellion and rejection are important ways of practicing sympathy and antipathy, as well as balance.

★ Young adolescents need healthy social and artistic outlets for giving expression to their newly strengthened world of feeling.

★ Style and individualized self-expression provide an outlet for those forces of emotion, and the exploration of new interests can provide much needed new orientation.

Transitions of self and identity

The last pair of developmental changes are perhaps less obvious and less well known, but they are just as important. Where birth and age 6–7 relate to physiologic processes of growth and thought, and 2–3 years and 12–14 years to experiences of emotion and social connection, 9 years and 20–21 years bring deeper experiences of self-identity.

9 years

When we reach all the way out through the circle of the twelve senses, the most outward sensing capacity we come to is the sense of 'I', the sense for engaging with another person's core individuality. Through this sense we see people on a deeper moral, even spiritual, level. That sensing really begins around age 9. The sense of 'I' becomes accessible at this time because it is the age when children take a big step in terms of feeling themselves on a core level.

During what is referred to as the '9-year-old change', each child finds connection to a richer experience of self. They realize that they are an individual being, a person completely distinct from anyone else. In anthroposophic medicine and Waldorf education this innermost aspect is known as the 'I' – because we can only say 'I' about ourselves. Age 9 marks an awakening of this innermost spiritual self, an awakening that may quietly also bring glimpses of key life themes and future intentions. This inner awakening of 'self' lays the foundation for greater moral perception, for a shift that starts with inner self-awareness and unfolds into an expanded, reciprocal understanding of the 'other'.

A prominent experience for many children at this age, however, is fear. 9-year-olds frequently express deep worries, and they tend to circle around particular themes: death, loss of a parent, illness, someone entering the house uninvited (robbers), car accidents, and natural disasters (like hurricanes, earthquakes, or tsunamis). These all are expressions of the newly experienced vulnerability that comes from feeling more separate, distinct and individual. When a child realizes that they are their own person, they also realize the potential for the loss of safety as well as the risk of losing those they love. The protective bubble of unconscious protection that shelters younger children thins as they wake up to more of the challenges and realities of the world.

This transition, more than almost any other developmental threshold, benefits from gentle companionship and courage.

It can indeed feel melancholy at times, but this stutter-step opens up into a fuller view of the individual beauty and originality of your child. As a society we really need to find better ways to actively celebrate and guide this shift in consciousness. As a physician I am always happy to meet and support children at this age because it marks a subtle but significant change, one which I learned nothing about in medical school and which is otherwise quite commonly misinterpreted. The '9-year-old change' opens a doorway to a new depth of meaning, morality, and courage when met in the right way.

What happens?

- ★ Children awaken to the fact that they are unique individuals who are separate from others (including parents, teachers, siblings, and relatives).
- ★ Instead of a big, outer physiologic shift, there is a deep inner change. Children's sphere of awareness – not of physical environment, but of self-identity – just took a big leap.
- ★ Nine-year-olds often develop fears: of illness, injury, death of a parent, crime, accidents, or natural disasters.
- ★ Children start to see how other people are also unique individuals, with unique qualities, feelings and quirks (like noticing how their parents are different than other parents, or that their teacher may have a life outside of school).
- ★ This sense of shifting orientation may even prompt some children to feel so independent, so newly separate, that

they may ask questions like, 'Where is my real family?' even if they are living with their birth parents in the home where they have always lived. The feeling of connectedness, which so naturally filled early childhood experiences, suddenly feels different.

★ Morality and fairness become an active part of their experience of the world.

What to do?

★ Realities of death, illness, separation, risk, can't so easily be tucked back in – the genie is well and truly out of the bottle. So merely discounting a child's worries does not fully reassure them. Acknowledgment becomes important: 'Yes, sometimes I worry about things too,' but that should also be combined with sharing about ways to work with it: 'If there were a tornado, we would go into the basement.' 'If we got in an accident, the doctors and nurses would help us get better.'

★ Be thoughtful about how much to share. Don't elaborate beyond a child's questions or concerns – they are still too young to share and know about all of your adult worries.

★ As with other periods of transition, rhythms are essential here too. Reassure your child that they do regular activities on a daily or weekly basis (eating, sleeping, going to school, seeing friends) because they are a normal part of life.

★ Too many options or decisions can create fatigue at this age, which often compounds underlying insecurities.

★ Help your child find ways to feel courage. Celebrate
successes and discoveries. Honor and welcome their
change. Who is this new person?

20-21 years

It might seem unusual to include this age in a listing of
children's biographical thresholds, but the end of the third
seven-year cycle marks a true end to childhood. Many young
adults go through an important time of reflection (sometimes
depression) during this year, as they move towards a further
step of self-perception.

The 21st year carries echoes of the 9-year-old change. What
was earlier an experience of oneself as a distinct individual,
now at around 20–21 years of age turns into a consideration
of what our individual path in life will be. We begin to take
an inner inventory, trying to balance patterns brought from
childhood with new, adult strivings for an independent
identity in the world. Self-orientation becomes connected to
finding one's own truth, and then finding the courage to give
that truth expression.

This process clearly does not end at 20–21 years. In fact,
this kind of emotional, social and spiritual inventory happens
quite predictably at the end of each seven-year cycle, at 27–28,
34–35, 41–42, 48–49, 55–56, 62–63, and beyond. Not every
seven-year cycle brings significant change for every person,
but there is a general truth that many people have made big
life changes during one or more of these windows of change.
Adult transitions, too, can have the quality of a stutter-step.

We invariably feel a bit wobbly in the process, but those wobbles are signs of ongoing developmental change and an opening into the next phase of growth.

What happens?

★ The true gateway into adulthood.
★ Each person actively seeks a new, independent experience of self, distinct from the family and community of childhood.
★ There is a readiness to more actively step out into one's own personal path of exploration and development.
★ This is a refinement and more conscious working with the experiences of individual self that first come around the age of 9.

What to do?

★ Honor the process.
★ Allow space for this kind of deep soul-searching to happen without worrying that something is terribly wrong with you or your life. You are right on time.
★ Seek the help and advice of others when you are feeling lost.
★ Remember that these biographical rhythms are potent times for growth, designed to bring a richer and more truthful sense of self.

AFTERWORD

What is the goal of sharing all this information? To help you work with the natural cycles and rhythms of sensory development in children. That development unfolds in time, much like the opening petals of a flower.

There is no obligation for you to follow any particular timing or schedule for any of these steps – just an invitation and an opportunity to see how learning about the inner sensory pathway can support children and help them better self-soothe, rest, connect to their sense of well-being, and develop greater resilience.

When we open a space for the evolving waves of sensory exploration and experience then we recognize, but perhaps no longer deeply fear, the stutter-steps along the way. For as a child expands and diversifies the ways they can feel 'well' in the world, they experience, more and more, 'What I need is right here.' That's a precious gift in this very busy world.

> Look for the goodness and
> capacity in your child.
> Trust in what is unfolding.
> Love your way through the stutter-steps.

ABOUT THE AUTHOR

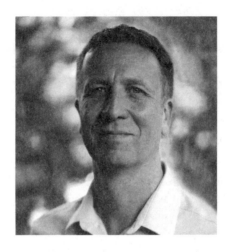

Dr Adam Blanning practices integrative and anthroposophic family medicine in Denver, Colorado. Alongside his work as a physician, Dr Blanning lectures and teaches internationally on topics relating to holistic medicine and the dynamics of human development, with a special interest in supporting children. He organizes training courses in anthroposophic medicine for physicians and other healthcare providers and works regularly with Steiner-Waldorf schools as a developmental consultant. Dr Blanning is a past president of the Anthroposophic Health Association (AHA) and the author of *Understanding Deeper Developmental Needs*, an in-depth exploration of challenging behaviors in children.

ENDNOTES

1. What Is the Inner Sensory Pathway?

1. Warmth has an unusual placement within the circle of the twelve senses – it is directed outward. A variety of research studies have explored the relationship between physical warmth and social perception, such as the fact that children on the autism spectrum more often show a decreased skin perception of warmth, but normal ranges of perception of pain. See https://pubmed.ncbi. nlm.nih.gov/25704841/ as an example.

2. Williams, L. E., 'Experiencing physical warmth promotes interpersonal warmth', *Science*. 2008 Oct. 24: 322(5901): 606–07. See https://pubmed.ncbi.nlm.nih.gov/18948544/

3. It is easiest to understand this progression with the example of listening to a foreign language. We might hear someone speak and not understand them. There are sounds, but at first they make no sense to us. Over time, as we slowly learn the language, we pick out the meaning of specific words. When we know enough words we can connect to someone's thoughts, and when we understand enough of another person's thoughts, we gain a deeper sense of their 'I', of their true individuality. Put differently, we may hear someone speak (in our own language), but not understand the words they are using; we may understand all the words, but be unable to connect to their thoughts; we may know their thoughts but only rarely find a connection to their true 'I'.

2: Soothing Patterns for Babies

1. Steiner, Rudolf, *Spiritual Science as a Foundation for Social Forms* (CW199), Anthroposophic Press, USA 1986, p. 39.
2. Nelson, Charles A. et al, *Romania's Abandoned Children: Deprivation, Brain Development, and the Struggle for Recovery.* Harvard University Press, USA 2014.

4: Finding Balance from Age 1 Onward

1. Steiner, Rudolf, *Spiritual Science as a Foundation for Social Forms* (CW199), p. 40.

7: Independence and Boundaries from Age 2½ Onward

1. Steiner, Rudolf, *Spiritual Science as a Foundation for Social Forms* (CW199), p. 40.

8: Building Well-being and Resilience for All Ages

1. Steiner, Rudolf, *Spiritual Science as a Foundation for Social Forms* (CW199), p. 42.
2. https://www.sleepfoundation.org/excessive-sleepiness/support/ how-much-sleep-do-babies-and-kids-need. Accessed June 3, 2020.
3. Campbell, W. Keith and Twenge, Jean M., 'Associations between screen time and lower psychological well-being among children and adolescents: Evidence from a population-based study', Campbell, *Preventive Medicine Reports* 12 (2008) 271–283.
4. You can find more information at the Harvard Center for the Developing child: https://developingchild.harvard.edu/resources/ aces-and-toxic-stress-frequently-asked-questions

9: Stuck Sensory Behaviors and Therapeutic Applications

1. It is common to wonder what normal or abnormal sexual behaviour in young children is, especially when they display unusual or unexpected interest in, or stimulation of, their genitals. Good resources include talking to your paediatrician or family doctor, plus websites like https://www.healthychildren.org/English/ages-stages/preschool/Pages/Sexual-Behaviours-Young-Children.aspx from the American Academy of Pediatrics. Accessed June 8, 2020.

10: Common Times of Anxiety and Transition

1. Selected milestones for gross motor, fine motor, language and social development Adapted from https://www.brightfutures.org/wellchildcare/toolkit/milestones/index.html, as well as the Denver II Developmental Screening test, https://doctorguidelines.com/2016/08/03/child-development-assessment-developmental-milestones-and-denver-developmental-screening-test/. Accessed on July 4, 2020.

2. For more information about sleep visit https://www.sleepfoundation.org/excessive-sleepiness/support/how-much-sleep-do-babies-and-kids-need and https://feedsleepbond.com/developmental-milestones-that-affect-sleep. Accessed on June 3, 2020.

3. For additional description of these rhythms in childhood, see *The First Seven Years: Physiology of Childhood*, Edmond Schoorel, Rudolf Steiner College Press, and descriptions of additional rhythms in adults life, see *Taking Charge: Your Life Patterns and Their Meaning*, Gudrun Burkhard, Floris Books, 1997.

4. Secondary sex characteristics come only at puberty, while primary sex characteristics are present at birth, meaning the presence of male or female genitalia.

ACKNOWLEDGMENTS

A book like this unfolds in many steps. The first was being born into a deeply loving and generous family. This book is dedicated to my parents, Nancy and Bill.

Then comes journeying, doctoring, collaborating, and parenting. Loving thanks go to my wife Lauren for all her support, and thanks to our children Eliza and Megan for joining us. You teach us new and wonderful things all the time. We are blessed.

Thanks also to Coco, Clair and Julie, key early readers of the book, and to the whole team at Floris Books for their wise guidance.

Lastly, to all the children who meet and seek the 'Toothpaste Treatment' – you are known and loved. May this book help you on your path.

A NOTE ON ANTHROPOSOPHIC MEDICINE

Anthroposophic medicine was founded in the 1920s by the philosopher and educator Rudolf Steiner and the physician Ita Wegman MD. It takes into account not just a person's physical and functional development, but also their emotional and spiritual health. It brings the same insights that stand behind Waldorf education into the realm of illness and healing. Natural, herbal and specially prepared medicines are offered to support, guide, or stimulate a new step in healing or development, and anthroposophic doctors, who are qualified MDs, work closely with teachers, therapists and parents to support healthy childhood. The gifts and perspectives this whole-person orientation provides feels timelier and ever more necessary in today's busy world.

To learn more:

- Physician's Association for Anthroposophic Medicine (PAAM), USA
  AnthroposophicMedicine.org

- Anthroposophic Medicine UK
  AnthroposophicMedicine.org.uk

- Australian Anthroposophic Medicine Association (AAMA), Australia
  Aamaanthro.com

- International Federation of Anthroposophic Medical Organizations (IVAA)
  IVAA.info

INDEX

You may also be interested in...

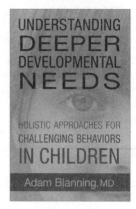

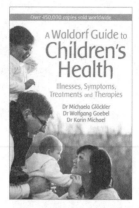

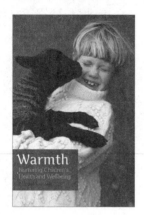

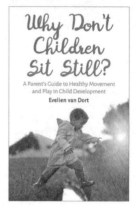

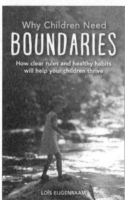

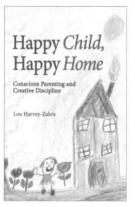

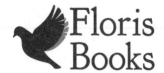

Floris
Books